Pathogenesis and Treatment of Chronic Pruritus

Pathogenesis and Treatment of Chronic Pruritus

Editor

Shawn G. Kwatra

MDPI • Basel • Beijing • Wuhan • Barcelona • Belgrade • Manchester • Tokyo • Cluj • Tianjin

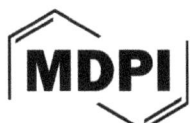

Editor
Shawn G. Kwatra
Johns Hopkins University School of Medicine
USA

Editorial Office
MDPI
St. Alban-Anlage 66
4052 Basel, Switzerland

This is a reprint of articles from the Special Issue published online in the open access journal *Medicines* (ISSN 2305-6320) (available at: https://www.mdpi.com/journal/medicines/special_issues/pathogenesis_chronic_pruritus).

For citation purposes, cite each article independently as indicated on the article page online and as indicated below:

LastName, A.A.; LastName, B.B.; LastName, C.C. Article Title. *Journal Name* **Year**, *Article Number*, Page Range.

ISBN 978-3-03943-100-7 (Hbk)
ISBN 978-3-03943-101-4 (PDF)

© 2020 by the authors. Articles in this book are Open Access and distributed under the Creative Commons Attribution (CC BY) license, which allows users to download, copy and build upon published articles, as long as the author and publisher are properly credited, which ensures maximum dissemination and a wider impact of our publications.

The book as a whole is distributed by MDPI under the terms and conditions of the Creative Commons license CC BY-NC-ND.

Contents

About the Editor .... **vii**

Kyle A. Williams and Shawn G. Kwatra
Emerging Research in Chronic Pruritus: From Bedside to Bench and Back Again
Reprinted from: *Medicines* **2020**, *7*, 24, doi:10.3390/medicines7050024 .... **1**

Katherine A. Whang, Raveena Khanna, Jamael Thomas, Crystal Aguh and Shawn G. Kwatra
Racial and Gender Differences in the Presentation of Pruritus
Reprinted from: *Medicines* **2019**, *6*, 98, doi:10.3390/medicines6040098 .... **7**

**Christina D. Kwon, Raveena Khanna, Kyle A. Williams, Madan M. Kwatra
and Shawn G. Kwatra**
Diagnostic Workup and Evaluation of Patients with Prurigo Nodularis
Reprinted from: *Medicines* **2019**, *6*, 97, doi:10.3390/medicines6040097 .... **15**

Katherine A. Whang, Sewon Kang and Shawn G. Kwatra
Inpatient Burden of Prurigo Nodularis in the United States
Reprinted from: *Medicines* **2019**, *6*, 88, doi:10.3390/medicines6030088 .... **25**

**John-Douglas Matthew Hughes, Taylor E. Woo, Micah Belzberg, Raveena Khanna,
Kyle A. Williams, Madan M. Kwatra, Shahzeb Hassan and Shawn G. Kwatra**
Association between Prurigo Nodularis and Etiologies of Peripheral Neuropathy: Suggesting
a Role for Neural Dysregulation in Pathogenesis
Reprinted from: *Medicines* **2020**, *7*, 4, doi:10.3390/medicines7010004 .... **35**

**Subuhi Kaul, Micah Belzberg, John-Douglas Matthew Hughes, Varun Mahadevan,
Raveena Khanna, Pegah R. Bakhshi, Michael S. Hong, Kyle A. Williams,
Annie L. Grossberg, Shawn G. Kwatra and Ronald J. Sweren**
Comorbidities in Mycosis Fungoides and Racial Differences in Co-Existent Lymphomatoid
Papulosis: A Cross-Sectional Study of 580 Patients in an Urban Tertiary Care Center
Reprinted from: *Medicines* **2020**, *7*, 1, doi:10.3390/medicines7010001 .... **45**

**Micah Belzberg, Valerie A. Larson, Raveena Khanna, Kyle A. Williams, Yevgeniy Semenov,
Sonja Ständer, Anna L. Grossberg and Shawn G. Kwatra**
Association between Itch and Cancer in 3836 Pediatric Pruritus Patients at a Tertiary
Care Center
Reprinted from: *Medicines* **2019**, *6*, 99, doi:10.3390/medicines6040099 .... **57**

**Amy H. Huang, Benjamin H. Kaffenberger, Adam Reich, Jacek C. Szepietowski,
Sonja Ständer and Shawn G. Kwatra**
Pruritus Associated with Commonly Prescribed Medications in a Tertiary Care Center
Reprinted from: *Medicines* **2019**, *6*, 84, doi:10.3390/medicines6030084 .... **67**

**Shawn G. Kwatra, Emily Boozalis, Amy H. Huang, Cory Nanni, Raveena Khanna,
Kyle A. Williams, Yevgeniy R. Semenov, Callie M. Roberts, Robert F. Burns,
Madison Krischak and Madan M. Kwatra**
Proteomic and Phosphoproteomic Analysis Reveals that Neurokinin-1 Receptor (NK1R)
Blockade with Aprepitant in Human Keratinocytes Activates a Distinct Subdomain of EGFR
Signaling: Implications for the Anti-Pruritic Activity of NK1R Antagonists
Reprinted from: *Medicines* **2019**, *6*, 114, doi:10.3390/medicines6040114 .... **75**

Akishi Momose, Micihihiro Yabe, Shigetoshi Chiba, Kenjirou Kumakawa, Yasuo Shiraiwa and Hiroki Mizukami
Role of Dysregulated Ion Channels in Sensory Neurons in Chronic Kidney Disease-Associated Pruritus
Reprinted from: *Medicines* **2019**, *6*, 110, doi:10.3390/medicines6040110 . . . . **83**

Michela Iannone, Agata Janowska, Valentina Dini, Giulia Tonini, Teresa Oranges and Marco Romanelli
Itch in Chronic Wounds: Pathophysiology, Impact, and Management
Reprinted from: *Medicines* **2019**, *6*, 112, doi:10.3390/medicines6040112 . . . . **91**

Ian P. Harrison and Fabrizio Spada
Breaking the Itch–Scratch Cycle: Topical Options for the Management of Chronic Cutaneous Itch in Atopic Dermatitis
Reprinted from: *Medicines* **2019**, *6*, 76, doi:10.3390/medicines6030076 . . . . **99**

Lisa L. Zhai, Kevin T. Savage, Connie C. Qiu, Annie Jin, Rodrigo Valdes-Rodriguez and Nicholas K. Mollanazar
Chronic Pruritus Responding to Dupilumab—A Case Series
Reprinted from: *Medicines* **2019**, *6*, 72, doi:10.3390/medicines6030072 . . . . **113**

Raveena Khanna, Emily Boozalis, Micah Belzberg, John G. Zampella and Shawn G. Kwatra
Mirtazapine for the Treatment of Chronic Pruritus
Reprinted from: *Medicines* **2019**, *6*, 73, doi:10.3390/medicines6030073 . . . . **129**

About the Editor

Shawn G. Kwatra is an Assistant Professor of Dermatology at the Johns Hopkins University School of Medicine. He is Director of the Johns Hopkins Itch Clinic and the Itch Fellowship Program. His areas of clinical expertise include chronic pruritus, prurigo nodularis, atopic dermatitis, and dermatology for ethnic skin. Dr. Kwatra's primary clinical and translational research interest is in the pathogenesis and treatment of chronic pruritus. He is supported by the Dermatology Foundation's Medical Dermatology Career Development Award.

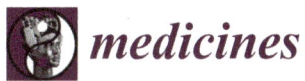

Editorial

Emerging Research in Chronic Pruritus: From Bedside to Bench and Back Again

Kyle A. Williams and Shawn G. Kwatra *

Department of Dermatology, Johns Hopkins University School of Medicine, Baltimore, MD 21287, USA; kwill223@jh.edu
* Correspondence: skwatra1@jhmi.edu; Tel.: +1-410-955-5933

Received: 21 April 2020; Accepted: 26 April 2020; Published: 29 April 2020

Abstract: This *Medicines* special issue highlights emerging research spanning from epidemiology to diagnostic workup, pathogenesis, and therapeutics for patients suffering from chronic pruritus. The special issue contains 13 articles reporting relevant epidemiologic and experimental data on chronic pruritus.

Keywords: pruritus; itch; treatment; therapeutic; pathogenesis; epidemiology

1. Introduction

This editorial serves as an introduction to the special issue "Pathogenesis and Treatment of Chronic Pruritus" and contains an overview of various known causes of chronic pruritus and emerging therapeutics. Chronic pruritus is itch that lasts greater than six weeks and is associated with a variety of dermatologic, systemic, neurologic, and psychiatric etiologies. Itch negatively impacts patient quality of life and has devastating psychosocial consequences. The manuscripts published in this special issue are also a showcase of the current understanding of the pathogenesis of chronic pruritus, along with its epidemiology, diagnostic workup, and therapeutic approaches used to treat chronic pruritus.

2. Epidemiology

Chronic pruritus can arise in association with many disease processes and affects many patient populations. Thus, epidemiologic studies are needed to gain a better understanding of the burden of disease. In this special issue, a cross-sectional study of over 18,000 itch patients seen at a tertiary care center showed that African American and female patients were more likely to experience pruritus than their white or male counterparts [1]. Furthermore, African American patients were less likely to see a dermatologist than other racial groups, suggesting disparities in care [1]. Additionally, African Americans were more likely to be diagnosed with prurigo nodularis (PN), lichen planus (LP), and atopic dermatitis (AD), which highlight areas for future translational studies. Finally, females were more likely to have comorbid autoimmune or psychiatric conditions [1]. This study's results were supported when their data was compared to nationally available data.

A major focus of this special issue is placed on prurigo nodularis. PN is a chronic itchy skin condition characterized by severely pruritic nodules that cause a significant negative impact on patient quality of life [2,3]. Kwon et al. performed a systematic review to provide a thorough testing and diagnostic evaluation algorithm for PN patients [4]. In particular, the study highlighted the need for baseline laboratory screening with complete blood cell count (CBC), complete metabolic panel (CMP), thyroid, liver, and kidney function tests, HIV serology, and hepatitis B and C serologies. Additional testing may be indicated based on individual patient's clinical history and review of systems [4].

Whang et al. sought to better characterize the epidemiology and disease burden of this condition by performing a cross-sectional study of the 2016 National Inpatient Sample [5]. Their study found that patients with PN accounted 3.7 inpatient visits per 100,000 discharges nationally [5]. Results also showed that patients diagnosed with PN were more likely to be African American or Asian, have longer and more costly hospital stays and be admitted for HIV complications [5]. These results are in line with prior studies on racial differences in prurigo nodularis [6].

Building on these findings, Hughes et al. conducted a cross-sectional analysis on the association of PN with various etiologies of peripheral neuropathy [7], and found significant associations with diabetes mellitus, chronic kidney disease (CKD), human influenza virus, metronidazole use, and hypothyroidism [7]. When compared to AD and psoriasis, the PN cohort was more likely to have chronic kidney disease and HIV [7].

Another skin condition featured in this special Issue is mycosis fungoides (MF). Patients with MF experience increased rates of cardiovascular disease and mortality when compared to healthy controls [8,9]. Recent studies have shown a relationship between MF and inflammatory disorders like psoriasis [9,10]. Given the chronic nature of this disease, comorbid conditions can significantly add to patient burden. Therefore, Kaul et al. performed a cross sectional study to evaluate 580 adult patients with diagnosed MF, to identify the common illnesses associated with MF and any racial differences in comorbid disease [11]. This study found that MF was strongly associated with lymphomatoid papulosis, Hodgkin's disease, congestive heart failure, hypertension, and hyperlipidemia compared with healthy controls [11]. Of note, the association between MF and lymphomatoid papulosis was seen in Caucasian and not African American patients [11]. The study provides valuable epidemiologic information on MF that can be used by clinicians managing this condition [11].

Malignancy is also associated with chronic pruritus [12,13]. The association between pruritus and cancer in adults is well recognized in the literature, in particular, with hematological malignancies such as Hodgkin's lymphoma, leukemia, and cutaneous T-cell lymphoma [13]. However, the prevalence of specific malignancy subtypes differ significantly between the pediatric and adult patient populations. Belzberg et al. performed a retrospective study to assess the association between pruritus and malignancy in pediatric patients [14]. This study found that pediatric patients with pruritus were 13 times more likely to have concomitant malignancy compared to pediatric patients without pruritus [14]. In the pediatric population, the correlation between pruritus and malignancy was strongest for cancers of the bone, skin, liver, and blood, as well as leukemia, non-Hodgkin's, and Hodgkin's lymphoma [14]. Pruritus may precede malignancy, concurrently appear, or also arise as a consequence of an adverse reaction of treatment [14].

Adverse drug reactions are also a well-recognized etiology of pruritus, and it has been shown by previous studies that pruritus accounts for over 10% of cutaneous drug reactions [15]. These adverse reactions can be chronic or acute and the pruritus generated can occur via direct skin inflammation or through systemic mediators depending on the causative drug [15]. In addition to the significant impact on quality of life pruritus can have, drug-induced pruritus also makes patients less compliant to their medication regimens [16]. Huang et al. performed a study to assess the rates of pruritus associated with commonly prescribed medications [16]. Using retrospective data of 9802 patients with pruritus after drug initiation, they found the highest rates of pruritus in patients taking heparin, trimethoprim-sulfamethoxazole, and calcium channel blockers [16]. They also found that of the pruritic patients a significantly larger proportion of them were female or African American [16].

Another class of medication known to be associated with drug induced pruritus are the Epidermal growth factor receptor (EGFR) inhibitors [17]. These medications, such as erlotinib, are often used as chemotherapeutic agents in cancer patients, but a recent survey showed that the cutaneous toxicities of these drug have led to clinicians having to adjust dosages and even discontinue them in patients experiencing these side effects [18]. One class of medications that have been suggested as a therapeutic agent for EGFR-associated pruritus are neurokinin-1 receptor (NK1R) antagonists [19]. Case series studies have reported efficacy in treating chronic itch with NK1R antagonists [20]. Additionally, a 2012 clinical trial supported the efficacy of the NK1R antagonists aprepitant in reducing pruritus caused by EGFR inhibitor therapy [21]. In an effort to better understand the antipruritic effect of aprepitant and its effect on human keratinocytes, Kwatra et al. performed reverse phase protein arrays (RPPA) to analyze its effect on these cells [22]. Results of this study found that aprepitant is a partial agonist of EGFR, and the researchers believe this action is responsible for its antipruritic effects [22]. This supports the need for further research on aprepitant as an itch fighting medication in vivo.

3. Pathophysiology

The pathophysiology of chronic pruritus is not yet fully understood but involves a complex interplay between the immune and neurologic systems and the skin [1]. As the pathogenesis of pruritus can differ based the etiology, this issue had multiple articles on itch subtypes. A systematic review was done to analyze current literature available on the characteristics and pathophysiological mechanisms of itch in chronic wounds [23]. This article suggested that a number of factors influence itch in chronic wounds including wound area, necrotic tissue amount, exudate amount, peripheral tissue edema, sclerosis, granulation tissue, perilesional skin characteristics, neuropathic changes, and dressing sensitization [23]. They also noted that there are currently no standards for preventing and managing itch in chronic wounds [23].

The relationship between nerve fibers and itch has been implicated in several pruritic conditions. Indeed, several itchy conditions have altered neural architecture as well as associated itch, and in some cases also an accompanying burning or pain sensations [24,25]. Chronic kidney disease-associated pruritus CKD-aP is thought to involve an alteration in nerve fibers and increased amounts of circulating pruritogens such as uremic toxins, which also stimulate reactive oxygen species (ROS) [26]. One study sought to further understand how the interact between uremic toxins and nerve fibers in patients with CKD-aP resulted in itch [27]. Momose et al. obtained skin biopsies from the forearm and elbow of two cohorts of patients. One group with CKD-aP and one with CKD patients not experiencing pruritus. After performing quantitative real-time polymerase chain reaction (RT-PCR) on these samples, the researchers found that the Cav3.2 T-type calcium channel, a channel only found in peripheral nerves of the skin that is associated with itch, was significantly higher in patients with CKD-aP than CKD patients without pruritus [27]. The researchers believe uremic toxins act on these ion channels in peripheral nerve endings and may serve as targets for future drugs to fight itch [27].

4. Treatment

With currently no U.S. Food and Drug Administration (FDA)-approved medications to specifically treat chronic itch as an indication, physicians are forced to use off label therapies [3]. Topical corticosteroid therapy has long been a first line therapy [28]. There are several additional topical agents used off label which Harrison et al. reviewed, including medications such as topical calcineurin inhibitors, capsaicin, ceramide, pine tar-based preparations, and doxepin [28].

The IL-4 receptor is another potential target for therapies aimed at alleviating chronic itch. IL-4 is believed to be a key upstream mediator of chronic pruritus associated with AD and downstream JAK signaling [29]. A case series published in this special issue reports significant itch improvement in a variety of pruritic conditions including, PN, LP, and uremic pruritus with dupilumab therapy [29].

Several antidepressants have also shown some benefits in treating itch [30–32]. Khanna et al. performed a systematic review to of the current literature to summarize the efficacy of mirtazapine, a tetracyclic antidepressant, in treating chronic itch [33]. The results suggest that mirtazapine may be an especially good option for recalcitrant itch in patients suffering from nocturnal itch who are underweight, as mirtazapine can cause sedation and weight gain.

In summary, our special issue highlights recent areas of clinical, translational, and basic science itch research. As itch has a significant effect on quality of life, it is our hope that these studies further stimulate research that may help contribute to the development of novel therapies for the treatment of chronic itch.

Author Contributions: K.A.W. and S.G.K. have contributed significantly and are in agreement with the content of the manuscript. All authors have read and agreed to the published version of the manuscript.

Funding: This article has no funding sources.

Conflicts of Interest: Shawn G. Kwatra is on the advisory board for Pfizer Inc., Regeneron Pharmaceuticals, and Menlo Therapeutics and has received grant funding from Kiniksa Pharmaceuticals. He is also the recipient of a Dermatology Foundation Medical Dermatology Career Development Award.

References

1. Whang, K.A.; Khanna, R.; Thomas, J.; Aguh, C.; Kwatra, S.G. Racial and Gender Differences in the Presentation of Pruritus. *Medicines* **2019**, *6*, 98. [CrossRef]
2. Huang, A.H.; Canner, J.K.; Khanna, R.; Kang, S.; Kwatra, S.G. Real-World Prevalence of Prurigo Nodularis and Burden of Associated Diseases. *J. Investig. Dermatol.* **2020**, *140*, 480–483.e4. [CrossRef]
3. Kwatra, S.G. Breaking the Itch–Scratch Cycle in Prurigo Nodularis. *N. Engl. J. Med.* **2020**, *382*, 757–758. [CrossRef] [PubMed]
4. Kwon, C.D.; Khanna, R.; Williams, K.A.; Kwatra, M.M.; Kwatra, S.G. Diagnostic Workup and Evaluation of Patients with Prurigo Nodularis. *Medicines* **2019**, *6*, 97. [CrossRef] [PubMed]
5. Whang, K.A.; Kang, S.; Kwatra, S.G. Inpatient Burden of Prurigo Nodularis in the United States. *Medicines* **2019**, *6*, 88. [CrossRef] [PubMed]
6. Boozalis, E.; Tang, O.; Patel, S.; Semenov, Y.R.; Pereira, M.P.; Stander, S.; Kang, S.; Kwatra, S.G. Ethnic differences and comorbidities of 909 prurigo nodularis patients. *J. Am. Acad. Dermatol.* **2018**, *79*, 714–719.e3. [CrossRef] [PubMed]
7. Hughes, J.D.M.; Woo, T.E.; Belzberg, M.; Khanna, R.; Williams, K.A.; Kwatra, M.M.; Hassan, S.; Kwatra, S.G. Association between Prurigo Nodularis and Etiologies of Peripheral Neuropathy: Suggesting a Role for Neural Dysregulation in Pathogenesis. *Medicines* **2020**, *7*, 4. [CrossRef] [PubMed]
8. Kim, Y.H.; Liu, H.L.; Mraz-Gernhard, S.; Varghese, A.; Hoppe, R.T. Long-term outcome of 525 patients with mycosis fungoides and Sézary syndrome: Clinical prognostic factors and risk for disease progression. *Arch. Dermatol.* **2003**, *139*, 857–866. [CrossRef] [PubMed]
9. Huang, A.H.; Kwatra, S.G.; Khanna, R.; Semenov, Y.R.; Okoye, G.A.; Sweren, R.J. Racial Disparities in the Clinical Presentation and Prognosis of Patients with Mycosis Fungoides. *J. Natl. Med. Assoc.* **2019**, *111*, 633–639. [CrossRef]
10. Nikolaou, V.; Marinos, L.; Moustou, E.; Papadavid, E.; Economidi, A.; Christofidou, E.; Gerochristou, M.; Tasidou, A.; Economaki, E.; Stratigos, A.; et al. Psoriasis in patients with mycosis fungoides: A clinicopathological study of 25 patients. *J. Eur. Acad. Dermatol. Venereol.* **2017**, *31*, 1848–1852. [CrossRef]
11. Kaul, S.; Belzberg, M.; Hughes, J.D.M.; Mahadevan, V.; Khanna, R.; Bakhshi, P.R.; Hong, M.S.; Williams, K.A.; Grossberg, A.L.; Kwatra, S.G.; et al. Comorbidities in Mycosis Fungoides and Racial Differences in Co-Existent Lymphomatoid Papulosis: A Cross-Sectional Study of 580 Patients in an Urban Tertiary Care Center. *Medicines* **2019**, *7*, 1. [CrossRef] [PubMed]
12. Larson, V.A.; Tang, O.; Ständer, S.; Kang, S.; Kwatra, S.G. Association between itch and cancer in 16,925 patients with pruritus: Experience at a tertiary care center. *J. Am. Acad. Dermatol.* **2019**, *80*, 931–937. [CrossRef] [PubMed]
13. Larson, V.A.; Tang, O.; Stander, S.; Miller, L.S.; Kang, S.; Kwatra, S.G. Association between prurigo nodularis and malignancy in middle-aged adults. *J. Am. Acad. Dermatol.* **2019**, *81*, 1198–1201. [CrossRef] [PubMed]
14. Belzberg, M.; Larson, V.A.; Khanna, R.; Williams, K.A.; Semenov, Y.; Ständer, S.; Grossberg, A.L.; Kwatra, S.G. Association between Itch and Cancer in 3836 Pediatric Pruritus Patients at a Tertiary Care Center. *Medicines* **2019**, *6*, 99. [CrossRef]
15. Reich, A.; Ständer, S.; Szepietowski, J.C. Drug-induced pruritus: A review. *Acta Derm. Venereol.* **2009**, *89*, 236–244. [CrossRef] [PubMed]
16. Huang, A.H.; Kaffenberger, B.H.; Reich, A.; Szepietowski, J.C.; Ständer, S.; Kwatra, S.G. Pruritus Associated with Commonly Prescribed Medications in a Tertiary Care Center. *Medicines* **2019**, *6*, 84. [CrossRef]
17. Kaul, S.; Kaffenberger, B.H.; Choi, J.N.; Kwatra, S.G. Cutaneous Adverse Reactions of Anticancer Agents. *Dermatol. Clin.* **2019**, *37*, 555–568. [CrossRef]

18. Hassel, J.C.; Kripp, M.; Al-Batran, S.; Hofheinz, R.-D. Treatment of Epidermal Growth Factor Receptor Antagonist-Induced Skin Rash: Results of a Survey among German Oncologists. *Onkologie* **2010**, *33*, 94–98. [CrossRef]
19. He, A.; Alhariri, J.M.; Sweren, R.J.; Kwatra, M.M.; Kwatra, S.G. Aprepitant for the Treatment of Chronic Refractory Pruritus. *Biomed Res. Int.* **2017**, *2017*, 4790810. [CrossRef]
20. Duval, A.; Dubertret, L. Aprepitant as an antipruritic agent? *N. Engl. J. Med.* **2009**, *361*, 1415–1416. [CrossRef]
21. Santini, D.; Vincenzi, B.; Guida, F.M.; Imperatori, M.; Schiavon, G.; Venditti, O.; Frezza, A.M.; Berti, P.; Tonini, G. Aprepitant for management of severe pruritus related to biological cancer treatments: A pilot study. *Lancet Oncol.* **2012**, *13*, 1020–1024. [CrossRef]
22. Kwatra, S.G.; Boozalis, E.; Huang, A.H.; Nanni, C.; Khanna, R.; Williams, K.A.; Semenov, Y.R.; Roberts, C.M.; Burns, R.F.; Krischak, M.; et al. Proteomic and Phosphoproteomic Analysis Reveals that Neurokinin-1 Receptor (NK1R) Blockade with Aprepitant in Human Keratinocytes Activates a Distinct Subdomain of EGFR Signaling: Implications for the Anti-Pruritic Activity of NK1R Antagonists. *Medicines* **2019**, *6*, 114. [CrossRef] [PubMed]
23. Iannone, M.; Janowska, A.; Dini, V.; Tonini, G.; Oranges, T.; Romanelli, M. Itch in Chronic Wounds: Pathophysiology, Impact, and Management. *Medicines* **2019**, *6*, 112. [CrossRef] [PubMed]
24. Mills, K.C.; Kwatra, S.G.; Feneran, A.N.; Pearce, D.J.; Williford, P.M.; D'Agostino, R.B.; Yosipovitch, G. Itch and pain in nonmelanoma skin cancer: Pain as an important feature of cutaneous squamous cell carcinoma. *Arch. Dermatol.* **2012**, *148*, 1422–1423. [CrossRef] [PubMed]
25. Bin Saif, G.A.; Alajroush, A.; McMichael, A.; Kwatra, S.G.; Chan, Y.H.; McGlone, F.; Yosipovitch, G. Aberrant C nerve fibre function of the healthy scalp. *Br. J. Dermatol.* **2012**, *167*, 485–489. [CrossRef] [PubMed]
26. Combs, S.A.; Teixeira, J.P.; Germain, M.J. Pruritus in Kidney Disease. *Semin. Nephrol.* **2015**, *35*, 383–391. [CrossRef]
27. Momose, A.; Yabe, M.; Chiba, S.; Kumakawa, K.; Shiraiwa, Y.; Mizukami, H. Role of Dysregulated Ion Channels in Sensory Neurons in Chronic Kidney Disease-Associated Pruritus. *Medicines* **2019**, *6*, 110. [CrossRef]
28. Harrison, I.P.; Spada, F. Breaking the Itch–Scratch Cycle: Topical Options for the Management of Chronic Cutaneous Itch in Atopic Dermatitis. *Medicines* **2019**, *6*, 76. [CrossRef]
29. Zhai, L.L.; Savage, K.T.; Qiu, C.C.; Jin, A.; Valdes-Rodriguez, R.; Mollanazar, N.K. Chronic Pruritus Responding to Dupilumab—A Case Series. *Medicines* **2019**, *6*, 72. [CrossRef]
30. Boozalis, E.; Khanna, R.; Zampella, J.G.; Kwatra, S.G. Tricyclic antidepressants for the treatment of chronic pruritus. *J. Dermatol. Treat.* **2019**, 1–3. [CrossRef]
31. Boozalis, E.; Khanna, R.; Kwatra, S.G. Selective serotonin reuptake inhibitors for the treatment of chronic pruritus. *J. Dermatol. Treat.* **2018**, *29*, 812–814. [CrossRef] [PubMed]
32. Boozalis, E.; Grossberg, A.L.; Püttgen, K.B.; Cohen, B.A.; Kwatra, S.G. Itching at night: A review on reducing nocturnal pruritus in children. *Pediatr. Dermatol.* **2018**, *35*, 560–565. [CrossRef] [PubMed]
33. Khanna, R.; Boozalis, E.; Belzberg, M.; Zampella, J.G.; Kwatra, S.G. Mirtazapine for the Treatment of Chronic Pruritus. *Medicines* **2019**, *6*, 73. [CrossRef] [PubMed]

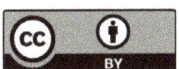

© 2020 by the authors. Licensee MDPI, Basel, Switzerland. This article is an open access article distributed under the terms and conditions of the Creative Commons Attribution (CC BY) license (http://creativecommons.org/licenses/by/4.0/).

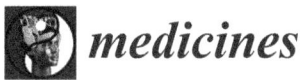

Article

Racial and Gender Differences in the Presentation of Pruritus

Katherine A. Whang [1], Raveena Khanna [1], Jamael Thomas [1,2], Crystal Aguh [1] and Shawn G. Kwatra [1,3,*]

[1] Department of Dermatology, Johns Hopkins University School of Medicine, Baltimore, MD 21231, USA; kwhang5@jhmi.edu (K.A.W.); rkhanna8@jhmi.edu (R.K.); jamael.thomas@utsouthwestern.edu (J.T.); cagi1@jhmi.edu (C.A.)
[2] School of Medicine, University of Texas Southwestern Medical Center, Dallas, TX 75390, USA
[3] Johns Hopkins Bloomberg School of Public Health, Baltimore, MD 21231, USA
* Correspondence: skwatra1@jhmi.edu; Tel.: +1-410-955-8662

Received: 27 June 2019; Accepted: 25 September 2019; Published: 27 September 2019

Abstract: Background: Pruritus is a common disease symptom with a variety of etiologies known to reduce patient quality of life. We aimed to characterize the racial and gender differences in the presentation of pruritus for itch-related patient visits both within a single institution and nationally. **Methods:** Cross sectional study of patients ≥ 18 years old seen at Johns Hopkins Health System between 1/1/12 and 1/1/18. Results were compared to data from 2005–2011 from the National Ambulatory Medical Care Survey (NAMCS) and the National Health Ambulatory Medical Care Survey (NHAMCS). **Results:** Our findings indicate that itch patients at JHHS (n = 18,753) were more likely to be black compared to white patients (37% vs. 19%, $p < 0.01$) when compared to patients without itch—a trend also noted nationally based on data from NAMCS/NHAMCS (26% vs. 21%, $p = 0.05$). Black itch patients are also more likely to be diagnosed with prurigo nodularis (OR 2.37, $p < 0.0001$), lichen planus (OR 1.22, $p < 0.0001$), and atopic dermatitis OR 1.51, $p < 0.0001$). Female itch patients are more likely to be diagnosed with autoimmune (OR 1.66, $p < 0.0001$) and psychiatric comorbidities (OR 1.2–1.8, $p < 0.0001$) than male itch patients. When compared to black itch patients nationally, white itch patients were more likely to visit a dermatologist (29% vs. 18%, $p = 0.028$). Our data can identify associated conditions and demographic differences but are unable to support a causal relationship. **Conclusions:** Black and female patients are more likely to present with pruritus, a symptom associated with comorbidities such as prurigo nodularis, lichen planus, atopic dermatitis, and psychiatric conditions.

Keywords: pruritus; itch; prurigo; nodularis; atopic; dermatitis; race; gender; comorbidities; demographics

1. Introduction

Pruritus is a common disease symptom known to negatively impact patient quality of life, contributing to both anxiety and depression. As a pervasive symptom, itch is present in an estimated 1% of all outpatient visits in the United States, occurring at any age and associated with a variety of dermatologic, systemic, neurologic, and psychiatric etiologies [1].

Pruritus arises from several different etiologies, from dermatoses and inflammation to infection, metabolic disease, cancer, psychiatric disease, drug application, and more. While the exact mechanism of pruritus is not fully understood, current evidence reveals the complex interplay between the skin, peripheral itch mediators such as histamine, neuropeptides, prostaglandins, and serotonin, and receptors, and the central nervous system. Sensation of itch, along with burning pain and heat, are transmitted through slow-conducting unmyelinated C-fibers. This pruritic information is thought to travel to the spinal cord via the dorsal root ganglion and travel along the spinothalamic tract [2]. Although histamine mediates a major itch pathway, non-histaminergic itch can be resistant to anti-histamine treatment and presents a challenge to clinicians.

Various different itch pathways have been implicated in different pruritic diseases. Atopic dermatitis (AD) is one example of a particularly pruritic dermatologic condition and is characterized by systemic epidermal barrier dysfunction. Increased transepidermal water loss, as commonly seen in AD, is highly associated with itch intensity [3]. Furthermore, the epidermal barrier dysfunction contributes to the entrance of irritants and pruritogens in AD patients, contributing to high pruritus burden. In contrast, psoriasis, which has been shown to have a lower burden of itch, is thought to be mediated by neurogenic inflammation and abnormal expression of neuropeptides such as substance P, calcitonin gene-related peptide, and somatostatin [4]. Studies have demonstrated that pruritus burden in psoriasis is associated with reduced health-related quality of life [5]. In terms of systemic causes of itch, pruritus due to cholestatic liver disease is believed to be due to pruritogens such as bile acids, lysophosphatidic acid, opiates, and progesterone derivatives [6].

Although gender and race are important factors in understanding disease etiology, there is limited knowledge on how these differences affect the presentation of pruritus. A 2013 study found that patients seen in visits for itch were more likely to be black or Asian than patients seen for other reasons [1]. Additionally, a German-based population study showed that women had higher visual analogue scale scores for itch severity, reported higher impact on quality of life, and presented with chronic scratch lesions more often than men, indicating gender-specific differences in underlying disease and burden among patients with chronic pruritus [7].

In our study, we sought to further understand the gender and racial differences in the presentation of pruritus by assessing itch-related patient visits in a tertiary care health system and national datasets.

2. Methods

Electronic health record system EPIC was used to collect anonymous aggregate-level retrospective data on patient demographics and comorbidities. We recorded the total number of patients age 18 years and older who had a chief complaint of "Pruritus" or a diagnosis of "Itching of the skin" from 1/1/12 to 1/1/18 using the systemized nomenclature of medicine—clinical terms (SNOMED-CT). Of these patients, we determined the percentage of patients with various dermatologic and non-dermatologic conditions known to be associated with pruritus and further stratified our results based on gender and race. Patient visits reporting itch were compared to controls, over the same time frame, of visits at JHHS that were not for itch. Odds ratios (ORs) were calculated to evaluate the strength of association of itch visits and diagnosis of various conditions when compared to the general patient population. Statistical significance was set at $p < 0.05$.

We also used data from the National Ambulatory Medical Care Survey (NAMCS) and the National Health Ambulatory Medical Care Survey (NHAMCS), nationally representative surveys conducted by the Centers for Disease Control and Prevention surveying office-based physicians, hospital emergency departments, and outpatient centers. Data from 2005–2011 were compiled to include entries for "Skin itching" in the "Reason for visit" field based on international classification of diseases—ninth revision, clinical modification (ICD-9-CM). The provided patient visit weights were applied to adjust for sampling probability and clustering effects and to determine nationally representative estimates of outpatient visits. Demographic and visit characteristics were compared between itch-related and non-itch-associated patient visits, for which a Pearson's chi-squared test was calculated to determine statistical significance. When adjusting for potential confounders such as age, sex, socioeconomic status, and region, an OR was generated by performing multivariable analysis using logistic regression.

3. Results

Table 1 shows the characteristics of visits for itch at JHHS and nationally, based on data from NAMCS/NHAMCS. Of the 18,753 patients seen for itch at JHHS, a greater percentage were female when compared to patients seen for other reasons (66% vs. 54%, $p = 0.01$). Patients seen for itch-related concerns were also more likely to be black (37% vs. 19%, $p < 0.01$) and Hispanic/Latino (5.8% vs. 2.7%, $p = 0.05$) when compared to patients without itch at JHHS. According to the national datasets, while a greater proportion of patients seen for pruritus were black (26% vs. 21%, $p = 0.05$), there were no other statistically significant differences in demographic characteristics in patients seen for itch complaints when compared to those without itch.

Table 1. Characteristics of visits for itch at JHHS (2012–2018) and the United Sates (2005–2011).

Demographics	JHHS			NAMCS		
	ITCH ($n = 18753$)	NO ITCH ($n = 4732084$)		ITCH ($n = 3778$)	NO ITCH ($n = 888990$)	
	% visits	% visits	p-value	% visits	% visits	p-value
Female	66.73	54.26	0.01	58.97	56.42	0.61
Male	31.17	45.45	0.01	41.03	43.58	0.61
Age						
Under 18 Years				17.05	20.15	0.44
18–24 Years	11.25	11.64	0.90	6.80	6.88	0.97
24–44 Years	28.29	28.23	0.99	18.79	22.71	0.35
45–64 Years	33.65	31.04	0.57	18.79	29.10	0.02
65–74 Years	16.18	14.29	0.59	6.01	10.78	0.12
75 Years and Older	10.62	14.79	0.24	6.48	10.37	0.20
Race						
White	47.82	54.18	0.20	65.38	73.99	0.05
Black	37.49	19.01	<0.01	25.62	20.65	0.05
Other	14.86	16.24	0.71	9.00	5.36	0.11
Ethnicity						
Hispanic or Latino	5.81	2.70	0.05	17.50	15.02	0.49
Not Hispanic or Latino	90.16	95.30	0.05	82.50	84.98	0.49

The data from JHHS were further utilized to assess racial differences in the percentage of itch patients who presented with various conditions commonly associated with pruritus symptoms. Of the patients seen for itch, blacks were more likely than whites to be diagnosed with atopic dermatitis (OR 1.51, $p < 0.0001$), lichen planus (OR 1.22, $p < 0.0001$), prurigo nodularis (OR 2.37, $p < 0.0001$), lichen simplex chronicus (OR 1.44, $p < 0.0001$), dry skin (OR 1.53, $p < 0.0001$), and systemic lupus erythematosus (OR 2.15, $p < 0.0001$) (Figure 1). In contrast, black patients seen for itch were less likely to present with psoriasis (OR 0.52, $p < 0.0001$), contact dermatitis (OR 0.82, $p < 0.0001$), stasis dermatitis (OR 0.57, $p < 0.0001$), and scalp pruritus (OR 0.89, $p < 0.0001$) when compared to white patients.

The differences in itch presentation can be explained by both physiologic variation and sociologic causes. To further explore the sociologic differences in pruritus presentation between black and white patients, we compared different visit characteristics in Figure 2 using NAMCS/NHAMCS datasets. Among the itch-related patients, more white patients had a history of a documented skin exam when compared to black patients (61% vs. 43%). Furthermore, white patients with itch symptoms were more likely to visit a dermatologist when compared to black patients with similar concerns, nationally (29% vs. 18%, OR 0.44, $p = 0.028$).

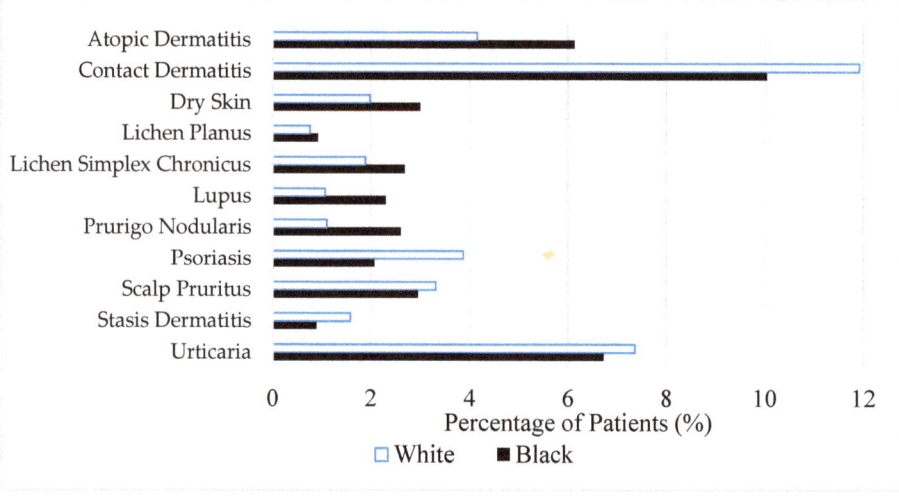

Figure 1. Percentage of white and black patients seen for itch diagnosed with various conditions.

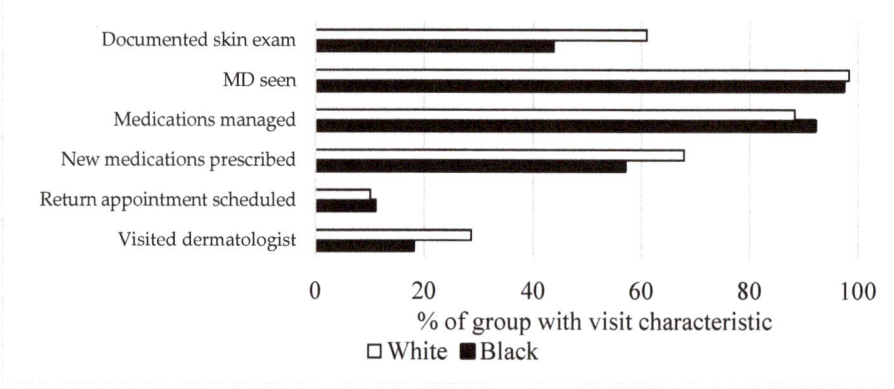

Figure 2. Visit characteristics for visits for itch nationally.

With regard to gender differences in the presentation of pruritus, females and males presented with different diagnoses for their itch symptoms at JHHS, as shown in Figure 3. Females reporting itch symptoms were more likely to be diagnosed with autoimmune conditions (OR 1.66, $p < 0.0001$), urticaria (OR 1.64, $p < 0.0001$), and sexually transmitted infections (OR 1.77, $p < 0.0001$) when compared to males reporting pruritus. However, women were less likely than men with itch to have kidney disease (OR 0.61, $p < 0.0001$), liver disease (OR 0.49, $p < 0.0001$), dermatophytes (0.59, $p < 0.0001$), or prurigo nodularis (0.61, $p < 0.0001$). Additionally, as shown in Figure 4, when investigating the prevalence of psychiatric comorbidities, both males and females suffering from pruritus were more likely to also be diagnosed with bipolar disorder, obsessive compulsive disorder, major depressive disorder, and generalized anxiety disorder when compared to the general patient population at JHHS (female: OR 7.1–9.6, $p < 0.0001$; male: OR 4.0–11.3, $p < 0.0001$). Of note, among the patients seen for pruritus, females are more likely than males to be diagnosed with these psychiatric comorbidities (OR 1.2–1.8, $p < 0.0001$).

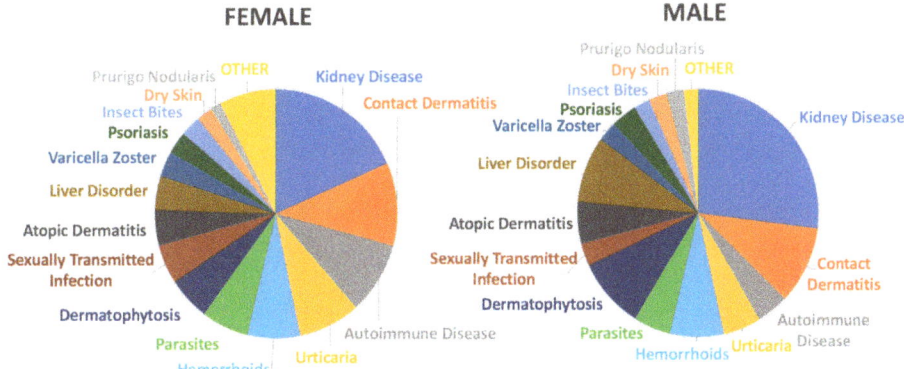

Figure 3. Gender differences in diagnosis.

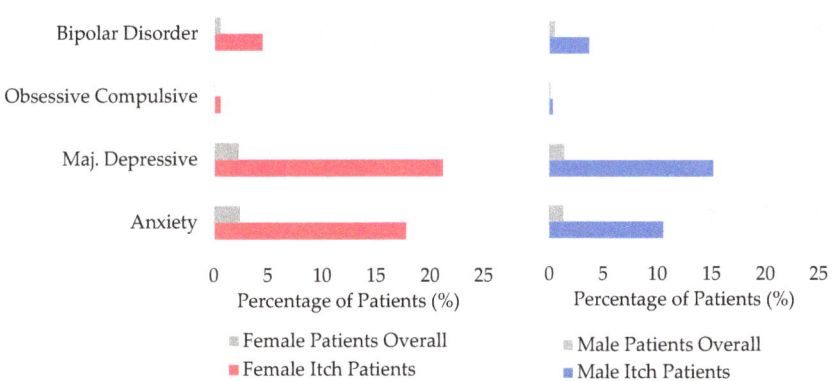

Figure 4. Comorbid psychiatric conditions in male and female pruritus patients compared to the general patient population at JHHS.

4. Discussion

This study characterized racial and gender differences in the presentation of pruritus at John Hopkins Health System and compared the results to those seen nationally. Our findings indicate that a greater proportion of black patients are affected by pruritus compared to white patients, and these patients are more likely to be diagnosed with certain dermatologic conditions including prurigo nodularis, lichen planus, and atopic dermatitis. However, black patients reporting itch symptoms are less likely to visit a dermatologist when compared to their white counterparts. Female itch patients are more likely to be diagnosed with autoimmune conditions and psychiatric comorbidities when compared to male itch patients.

Despite the fact that patients with itch symptoms at JHHS were more likely to be female, black, and Hispanic or Latino, assessment of the national patient population partially confirmed these findings; a greater proportion of pruritus patients were black than non-pruritus patients, but there were not significant gender differences.

This study reports the increased risk in black itch patients for atopic dermatitis, dry skin, SLE, prurigo nodularis, lichen planus, and lichen simplex chronicus. While previous research has described these racial differences in atopic dermatitis and SLE, there is very little epidemiologic data on prurigo nodularis, lichen planus, and lichen simplex chronicus. Studies at our institution demonstrated that prurigo nodularis disproportionately affects black patients [8,9]. Our group also recently confirmed that PN disproportionately affects blacks and Asians in nationwide studies [10–12]. Our results indicating racial differences in the prevalence of certain dermatologic conditions can be attributed to the physiologic variation of skin between the races. For example, black skin has been found to have a lower pH, lower ceramide content within the stratum corneum, greater cohesion between keratinocytes and increased mast cells [13]. Knowledge of these differences and how they affect presentation of dermatologic symptoms such as pruritus can help guide treatment.

Despite the fact that black patients are more likely to report pruritus, we observed that even when adjusting for age, sex, socioeconomic status, and region, black itch patients were less likely to visit a dermatologist than white itch patients. Similarly, a study on the treatment of acne vulgaris demonstrated that black acne patients were less likely to visit a dermatologist than white acne patients [14]. Further research is necessary to validate these findings and better understand the cause for these disparities in the access and utilization of care.

In addition to the racial differences, there are several gender differences, as seen in Figures 3 and 4, that may contribute to our understanding of pruritic symptoms. While autoimmune conditions, urticaria, and sexually transmitted infections are more likely to be associated with pruritus in females, liver and kidney disease, dermatophytosis, and prurigo nodularis are more likely to be diagnosed in males with pruritus. Many of these differences can be attributed to the epidemiology of the conditions themselves. Autoimmune conditions and urticaria both occur more commonly in women, perhaps because of differences in sex hormones and inflammation pathways, which are reflected in our findings [15]. Women are found to progress toward end-stage renal disease at a slower rate than men, thus explaining the gender discrepancy in pruritic presentation with kidney disease [16].

Although the exact pathophysiology of pruritus is not fully elucidated, the central neural mechanisms of itch have been suggested to be mediated by neuropeptides, especially endogenous opioids, and histamine [17,18]. Gupta et al. described the association between depression and elevated levels of corticotropin releasing factor, leading to increased central opiate levels and heightened perception of itch sensation [19]. Here, the increased risk of psychiatric comorbidities in all pruritus patients when compared to the general patient population underscores the strong central component of pruritus. Furthermore, women reporting pruritus symptoms are more likely than males to have comorbid psychiatric conditions. Studies of patients with chronic pruritus have shown that women have higher anxiety scores and levels of neuropathic and psychosomatic disease, which is in accordance with our findings [7]. Knowledge of the increased prevalence of psychiatric comorbidities in patients reporting pruritus will help providers better manage pruritic dermatologic disease.

Overall, even though itch is a common symptom in many diseases, there is little knowledge about the influence of gender and race in pruritus. Our study illustrates both gender and racial differences in the presentation of patients with pruritus symptoms. Future studies should investigate the causes of such differences and to address these disparities.

Author Contributions: K.A.W., R.K., and S.G.K. had full access to all of the data in the study and take responsibility for the integrity of the data and accuracy of the data analysis. Conceptualization, K.A.W. and S.G.K.; Methodology, K.A.W. and S.G.K.; Software, K.A.W. and S.G.K.; Validation, K.A.W. and S.G.K.; Formal Analysis, K.A.W.; Investigation, K.A.W., R.K. and S.G.K.; Resources, S.G.K.; Data Curation, K.A.W., R.K., J.T., C.A., and S.G.K.; Writing—Original Draft Preparation, K.A.W. and S.G.K.; Writing-Review & Editing, J.T. and C.A.; Visualization, K.A.W., R.K., S.G.K.; Supervision, S.G.K.; Project Administration, S.G.K.

Funding: This research received no external funding.

Conflicts of Interest: Shawn G. Kwatra is on the advisory board and serves as a consultant for Menlo Therapeutics, and has received grant funding from Kiniksa Pharmaceuticals. He is also a recipient of a Dermatology Foundation Medical Dermatology Career Development Award. The other author(s) have no conflict of interest to declare.

References

1. Shive, M.; Linos, E.; Berger, T.; Wehner, M.; Chren, M.-M. Itch as a patient-reported symptom in ambulatory care visits in the United States. *J. Am. Acad. Dermatol.* **2013**, *69*, 550–556. [CrossRef] [PubMed]

2. Ständer, S.; Steinhoff, M.; Schmelz, M.; Weisshaar, E.; Metze, D.; Luger, T. Neurophysiology of Pruritus: Cutaneous Elicitation of Itch. *Arch. Dermatol.* **2003**, *139*, 1463–1470. [CrossRef] [PubMed]
3. Lee, C.; Chuang, H.; Shih, C.; Jong, S.; Chang, C.; Yu, H. Transepidermal water loss, serum IgE and b-endorphin as important and independent biological markers for development of itch intensity in atopic dermatitis. *Br. J. Dermatol.* **2006**, *154*, 1100–1107. [CrossRef] [PubMed]
4. Szepietowski, J.C.; Reich, A. Pruritus in psoriasis: An update. *Eur. J. Pain* **2016**, *20*, 41–46. [CrossRef] [PubMed]
5. Mrowietz, U.; Chouela, E.N.; Mallbris, L.; Stefanidis, D.; Marino, V.; Pedersen, R.; Boggs, R.L. Pruritus and quality of life in moderate-to-severe plaque psoriasis: Post hoc explorative analysis from the PRISTINE study. *Eur. Acad. Dermatol. Venereol.* **2015**, *29*, 1114–1120. [CrossRef] [PubMed]
6. Patel, S.; Vasavda, C.; Ho, B.; Meixiong, J.; Dong, X.; Kwatra, S. Cholestatic pruritus: Emerging mechanisms and therapeutics. *J. Am. Acad. Dermatol.* **2019**, *2019*. [CrossRef] [PubMed]
7. Ständer, S.; Stumpf, A.; Osada, N.; Wilp, S.; Chatzigeorgakidis, E.; Pfleiderer, B. Gender differences in chronic pruritus: Women present different morbidity, more scratch lesions and higher burden. *Br. J. Dermatol.* **2013**, *168*, 1273–1280. [CrossRef] [PubMed]
8. Boozalis, E.; Tang, O.; Patel, S.; Semenov, Y.R.; Pereira, M.P.; Stander, S.; Kang, S.; Kwatra, S.G. Ethnic differences and comorbidities of 909 prurigo nodularis patients. *J. Am. Acad. Dermatol.* **2018**, *79*, 714–719. [CrossRef] [PubMed]
9. Bender, A.M.; Tang, O.; Khanna, R.; Ständer, S.; Kang, S.; Kwatra, S.G. Racial differences in dermatological conditions associated with Human Immunodeficiency Virus: A cross-sectional study of 4,679 patients in an urban tertiary care center. *J. Am. Acad. Dermatol.* **2019**, *2019*. [CrossRef] [PubMed]
10. Whang, K.A.; Kang, S.; Kwatra, S.G. Inpatient Burden of Prurigo Nodularis in the United States. *Medicines* **2019**, *6*, 88. [CrossRef] [PubMed]
11. Huang, A.H.; Canner, J.K.; Kang, S.; Kwatra, S.G. Analysis of real-world treatment patterns in patients with prurigo nodularis. *J. Am. Acad. Dermatol.* **2019**, *2019*. [CrossRef] [PubMed]
12. Huang, A.H.; Canner, J.K.; Khanna, R.; Kang, S.; Kwatra, S.G. Real-world prevalence of prurigo nodularis and burden of associated diseases. *J. Investig. Dermatol.* **2019**, *2019*. [CrossRef] [PubMed]
13. Czerkasij, V. Skin of color. *Nurse Pract.* **2013**, *38*, 34–40. [CrossRef] [PubMed]
14. Rogers, A.T.; Semenov, Y.R.; Kwatra, S.G.; Okoye, G.A. Racial disparities in the management of acne: Evidence from the National Ambulatory Medical Care Survey, 2005–2014. *J. Dermatolog. Treat.* **2018**, *29*, 287–289. [CrossRef] [PubMed]
15. Fairweather, D.; Frisancho-Kiss, S.; Rose, N.R. Sex Differences in Autoimmune Disease from a Pathological Perspective. *Am. J. Pathol.* **2008**, *173*, 600–609. [CrossRef] [PubMed]
16. Cobo, G.; Hecking, M.; Port, F.K.; Exner, I.; Lindholm, B.; Stenvinkel, P.; Carrero, J.J. Sex and gender differences in chronic kidney disease: progression to end-stage renal disease and haemodialysis. *Clin. Sci.* **2016**, *130*, 1147–1163. [CrossRef] [PubMed]
17. Lee, H.G.; Stull, C.; Yosipovitch, G. Psychiatric disorders and pruritus. *Clin. Dermatol.* **2017**, *35*, 273–280. [CrossRef] [PubMed]
18. Jafferany, M.; Davari, M.E. Itch and psyche: Psychiatric aspects of pruritus. *Int. J. Dermatol.* **2019**, *58*, 3–23. [CrossRef] [PubMed]
19. Gupta, M.; Gupta, A.; Schork, N.; Ellis, C. Depression modulates pruritus perception: A study of pruritus in psoriasis, atopic dermatitis, and chronic idiopathic urticaria. *Psychosom. Med.* **1994**, *56*, 36–40. [CrossRef] [PubMed]

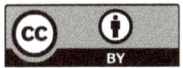

© 2019 by the authors. Licensee MDPI, Basel, Switzerland. This article is an open access article distributed under the terms and conditions of the Creative Commons Attribution (CC BY) license (http://creativecommons.org/licenses/by/4.0/).

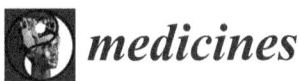

Communication

Diagnostic Workup and Evaluation of Patients with Prurigo Nodularis

Christina D. Kwon [1,*], Raveena Khanna [1], Kyle A. Williams [1], Madan M. Kwatra [2] and Shawn G. Kwatra [1]

[1] Department of Dermatology, Johns Hopkins University School of Medicine, Baltimore, MD 21231, USA; rkhanna8@jhmi.edu (R.K.); Kwill184@health.fau.edu (K.A.W.); skwatra1@jhmi.edu (S.G.K.)
[2] Department of Anesthesiology, Duke University School of Medicine, Durham, NC 27710, USA; kwatr001@mc.duke.edu
* Correspondence: ckwon18@jhmi.edu; Tel.: +1-281-777-4172

Received: 1 August 2019; Accepted: 23 September 2019; Published: 26 September 2019

Abstract: Prurigo nodularis (PN) is a chronic inflammatory skin disease characterized oftentimes by symmetrically distributed, severely pruritic nodules. Currently, the pathophysiology of PN remains to be fully elucidated, but emerging evidence suggests that neuroimmune alterations play principal roles in the pathogenesis of PN. There are several associated etiologic factors thought to be associated with PN, including dermatoses, systemic, infectious, psychiatric, and neurologic conditions. We conducted a systematic literature review to evaluate the clinical presentation, diagnosis, and etiologic factors of PN. In this review, we discuss common differential diagnoses of PN and recommend an evidence-based, standardized diagnostic evaluation for those with suspected PN.

Keywords: medical dermatology; prurigo nodularis; systematic review; itch; pruritus

1. Introduction

Prurigo nodularis (PN) is a chronic inflammatory skin disease characterized oftentimes by symmetrically distributed, severely pruritic nodules. Currently, the pathophysiology of PN remains to be fully elucidated, but emerging evidence suggests that neuroimmune alterations play principal roles in the pathogenesis of PN. PN is also associated with several disease comorbidities such as chronic renal failure, liver disease, HIV, and malignancy [1–4]. However, there are currently no FDA approved therapies for PN, and patients are often times recalcitrant to off-label therapies. The goal of the present study is to perform a systematic review in the literature to provide evidence for specific testing and diagnostic evaluation of PN patients.

2. Methods

Using the Preferred Reporting Items for Systematic Reviews and Meta-Analyses (PRISMA) guidelines, we searched the PubMed, MEDLINE and Embase databases for "prurigo nodularis" or "prurigo." All articles, including case reports and series describing prurigo nodularis were included. English language articles were included before April 8, 2019. We limited the search to articles involving human subjects. All of the results were checked for relevance and suitability. No manufacturers or authors mentioned in these reports were contacted.

3. Results

Our search yielded a total of 791 records with redundancy from 1947 to 2019 containing the aforementioned key words. After removing duplicates, 342 unique records remained. Ultimately, 35 primary sources were included. We included case series and reports. In these sources, the clinical presentation, potential pathophysiology, histological characteristics and etiologic factors of PN were discussed.

4. Diagnosis

4.1. History and Physical

PN is a clinical diagnosis that is based upon information gathered from a thorough history and physical examination. In regard to history, patients will complain of severe itch that can be continuous, paroxysmal or sporadic. In addition to pruritus, patients may also describe the sensations as a burning or stinging [5].

PN characteristically presents with excoriated, hyperkeratotic, and pruritic dome-shaped nodules, papules, or plaques that are often bilaterally distributed on the extensor surfaces of the extremities (Figure 1) [6]. In addition to affecting extremities, PN can also involve parts of the trunk that are accessible to scratching such as the upper back and abdomen. Patients with back involvement often present with the "butterfly" sign as they are unable to reach the central back and this area is spared, leaving a characteristic butterfly pattern [7]. The lesions can be variable in both quantity and quality. Cases range from patients having only a few lesions to several hundreds. The lesions also vary in size, from millimeters to centimeters, and color, ranging from flesh-colored to pink to brown or black.

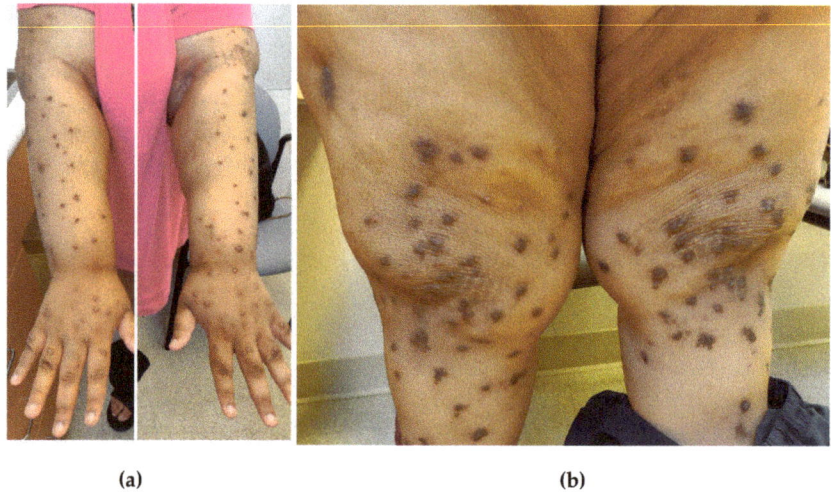

(a) (b)

Figure 1. (a) Nodules in bilateral distribution on arms and (b) legs in a patient diagnosed with prurigo nodularis.

4.2. Differential Diagnoses

There are several skin diseases that can mimic PN. We discuss several rare conditions that have been reported in the literature as being masqueraders of PN. Often, these diagnoses are only elucidated after the patient is refractory to treatment and worked-up further.

4.2.1. Pemphigoid Nodularis

Pemphigoid nodularis is a rare variant of bullous pemphigoid that has features of both prurigo nodularis and bullous pemphigoid. Compared to PN, pemphigoid nodularis is often characterized by larger plaques often with large areas of central erosion, ulceration, and/or blistering [8,9]. On biopsy, there is also evidence of subepidermal clefting and direct immunofluorescence (DIF) displays linear deposition of IgG and C3 at the basement membrane zone. Furthermore, patients will have circulating antibasement membrane zone autoantibodies [10–12].

4.2.2. Actinic Prurigo

Actinic prurigo is a rare type of photodermatosis presenting with acute eruptions of severely pruritic papules or nodules often accompanied by cheilitis and conjunctivitis. This condition is more common in young girls and they present with extreme photosensitivity to UVA and UVB [13].

4.2.3. Epidermolysis Bullosa

Epidermolysis bullosa (EB) has multiple variants such as EB pruriginosa and acquista that can sometimes present with nodular prurigo-like lichenified lesions seen in PN [14]. Diagnosis is often based on immunofluorescence showing antibodies against type VII collagen in the sublamina densa [15].

4.2.4. Hypertrophic Lichen Planus

Hypertrophic lichen planus (HLP) can also resemble PN clinically, presenting as hyperkeratotic plaques and nodules most commonly involving the shin and ankles. Histopathology can also be very similar with both demonstrating epidermal hyperplasia, hypergranulosis, compact hyperkeratosis, increased number of fibroblasts and capillaries. However, basal cell degeneration is confined to the tips of the rete ridges and band-like infiltration is often absent in HLP compared to PN [16].

4.2.5. Neurotic Excoriations

Neurotic excoriations, also known as dermatotillomania, can also lead to excoriations that can have slightly raised areas that resemble lesions seen in PN. Neurotic excoriations, however, is a psychiatric condition characterized by excessive picking of the skin.

Lastly, some more common differential diagnoses to consider include the following: insect bites, scabies surrepticius, lupus erythematosus, multiple keratoacanthomas, atopic dermatitis, and psoriasis vulgaris [17,18].

5. Etiologic Factors and Associated Diseases

5.1. Dermatoses

Some studies have pointed to dermatological conditions as the predominant etiology of PN, up to 82% [5,19]. PN has been associated with a variety of dermatological conditions, most notably atopic dermatitis (up to 46%) [5,19–22]. Other dermatological conditions that have been associated with PN are cutaneous T-cell lymphoma, lichen planus, xerosis cutis, keratoacanthomas, and bullous pemphigoid [5,23,24]. One study found that 60% of its cohort of patients with PN ($n = 80$) had xerosis. In these patients with xerosis, there were higher rates of co-morbidities including diabetes and psychiatric causes, which is discussed below [21].

5.2. Systemic

Systemic and metabolic causes have been implicated in 38% to up to 50% of PN cases [25,26]. Some common systemic associations of PN are chronic renal failure, liver disease (chronic hepatitis B, primary biliary cholangitis, chronic autoimmune cholestatic hepatitis), HIV, thyroid disease, diabetes and malignancies, specifically non-Hodgkin's lymphoma [3,4,27–36]. A study ($n = 16,925$) by Larson et al. found that pruritus was most strongly associated with cancers of the liver, skin, and hematopoietic system [37]. Rarer malignancies that have been associated with PN are metastatic transitional cell carcinoma of the bladder and Hodgkin's lymphoma [30,38,39]. Other less commonly associated systemic causes are gout, iron-deficiency anemia, and celiac disease [26,32,40,41].

5.3. Infectious

A number of infectious causes have been implicated in PN [42]. Some infectious or parasitic causes that have been reported are *Mycobacterium tuberculosis* and *mucogenicum*, *Ascaris lumbricoides*, *Helicobacter pylori*, *Strongyloides stercoralis*, and herpes zoster [42–50]. In some cases, it has been found that treatment and resolution of the infection have resolved the PN and pruritic symptoms. Although the aforementioned studies and reports have linked infectious agents with PN, there is still a lack of strong evidence for a direct causal association [42].

5.4. Medications

Medications have been reported as a cause of PN. There have been reports implicating mainly cancer therapy agents in cutaneous side effects [48,49]. In a study by Biswal et al., 384 out of 1000 patients undergoing chemotherapy developed cutaneous adversities. Of the 384, 0.8% ($n = 3$) developed prurigo nodularis [51]. Specifically, pembrolizumab, paclitaxel, and carboplatin have been associated with the development of PN [51,52]. With these therapy agents it is thought that the persistent activation of the immune system contributes to the pathogenesis of PN. For example, pembrolizumab is an antibody that works as an immune checkpoint inhibitor by blocking programmed death 1 protein.

5.5. Psychiatric

PN has been significantly associated with depression, anxiety, and dissociative experiences, all of which can cause psychogenic pruritus [1,53–58]. This psychogenic pruritus is then thought to lead to PN. However, psychogenic pruritus must be distinguished from neurotic excoriations (also known as dermatotillomania), which is characterized by excessive scratching or picking of the skin, leading to skin lesions. Of note, dermatotillomania is categorized as an impulse disorder and is frequently associated with other primary psychiatric impulse disorders [59].

5.6. Neurologic

Neuropathic itch is a pathological condition due to some neuronal or glial damage. It has many causes including local nerve fiber compression or degeneration. Although it is more common to involve the peripheral nervous system (PNS), neuropathic itch can also stem from damage within the central nervous system (CNS) [60]. Proximal PNS etiologies are polyneuropathies, post-herpetic neuralgia, brachioradial pruritus, notalgia paraesthetica, and other entrapment neuropathies [61]. Distal PNS etiologies include small-fiber neuropathies, sensitive skin, or post-burn itch [61].

6. Evaluation

6.1. Biopsy

Although PN is a clinical diagnosis, biopsies are often warranted for lesions that do not respond to first line therapies or those with secondary complications such as bleeding or ulceration. Weigelt et al. found that PN ($n = 136$) had characteristic features such as presence of thick orthohyperkeratotis, the hairy palm sign (folliculosebaceous units seen with a thick and compact cornified layer), irregular epidermal hyperplasia, hypergranulosis, fibrosis of the papillary dermis and increased fibroblasts and capillaries. However, these histologic characteristics often coincide with other scratch-induced conditions, such as lichen simplex. Thus, correlation of clinical and histological findings is still required to distinguish PN from other scratched-induced conditions [62].

Immunohistochemical studies have shown reduced intraepidermal nerve fiber density in lesional and nonlesional skin in patients with prurigo nodularis [63]. This observed hypoplasia has been suggested to indicate subclinical small fiber neuropathy PN [63]. However, recent studies have shown that there is no functional small fiber-neuropathy and the altered epidermal neuroanatomy is thought to be a consequence of chronic scratching [64]. As a result, we do not currently recommend routine intraepidermal nerve fiber density (IENFD) testing in patients unless underlying small fiber neuropathy is suspected. Direct immunofluorescence (DIF) is helpful for distinguishing PN from autoimmune diseases, such as bullous pemphigoid, pemphigoid nodularis, and epidermolysis bullosa, which may present similarly, or even concomitantly, with PN [23].

6.2. Laboratory Evaluation

As previously mentioned, PN can often have an associated systemic etiology. A thorough laboratory work-up should be pursued, especially for patients without a history of underlying dermatoses, such as PN arising secondary to atopic dermatitis. Systemic causes of chronic pruritus should be particularly evaluated for common systemic etiologies, such as chronic renal failure, liver disease, HIV, and thyroid disease. Infrequently, PN has presented in the context of gout, iron-deficiency anemia, celiac disease, non-Hodgkin's lymphoma or infection.

Strongly suggested workup includes a complete blood cell count (CBC), complete metabolic panel (CMP), thyroid, liver and kidney function tests, HIV serology, and hepatitis B and C serologies (Figure 2). Optional workup based on clinical judgement and the patient's clinical examination includes biopsy with a hematoxylin and eosin stain, direct immunofluorescence, chest radiograph, serum and urine protein electrophoresis, urinalysis, stool exam for ova and parasites, and iron studies.

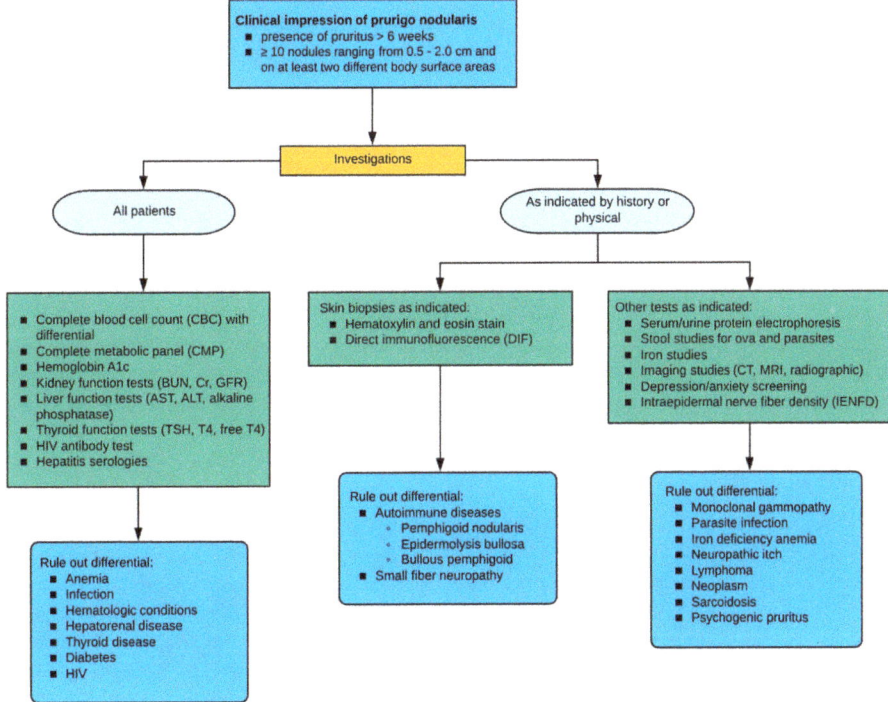

Figure 2. Diagnostic approach and workup for patients with prurigo nodularis.

6.3. Pruritic Intensity and Quality of Life

In addition to the above, evaluation should also take pruritic symptoms and quality of life into consideration given the severe pruritus that PN patients often experiences [65]. There is a wide range of different scales that have been used to assess pruritic symptoms. In terms of pruritic intensity, there are monodimensional tools that have shown high reliability and concurrent validity, such as the

Visual Analogue Scale (VAS), Itch Numerical Rating Scale (Itch NRS), Worst Itch Numeric Rating Scale (WI-NRS), and Verbal Rating Scale (VRS) [65,66]. The VAS uses a 10 cm scale with endpoints marked with "0" and "10" to correlate with "no itch" and "worst imaginable itch," respectively [65]. With the NRS, patients are asked to rate their itch intensity from 0 for "no itch" to 10 for "worst imaginable itch." Lastly, the VRS asks patients to describe their itch symptom intensity with a list of adjectives such as "0 = no itch" and "1 = mild itch" [67].

There are also multidimensional scales to assess pruritus intensity. These include the Itch Severity Scale (ISS) and the Pruritus Grading System (PGS). These multidimensional scales encompass questions around the time of day pruritic symptoms occur, the quality, intensity and location of itch, and effects on sexual symptom and sleep [68].

In terms of assessing scratch activity and lesions, there are tools available such as the Scratch Symptom Score (SSS), Prurigo Activity Score (PAS), wrist actigraphy, and accelerometers. The SSS measures individual scratch lesions standardized against the body surface [65]. The PAS is a seven-item questionnaire designed to monitor the distribution and activity of chronic prurigo lesions [69]. Although wrist actigraphy and accelerometers may prove useful in assessing activity, they have yet to be validated and may not be easily conducted in a clinic setting [65,70].

In addition to the above scales and questionnaires that often capture a patient's itch symptoms at one point in time, there are also several tools available to monitor the course of pruritus. These include: the Dynamic Pruritus Score, Itch-Free Days, 5-D Itch Scale, Patient Benefit Index, and ItchApp [65]. These various tools encompass the course of itch intensity and location, patient satisfaction with treatment, changing symptoms and disability over different points in time.

As previously mentioned, there are high rates of psychiatric comorbidities associated with PN. Some tools used to assess depression and anxiety include: the Beck Depression Inventory, Hospital Anxiety and Depression Scale, and Hamilton Rating Scale for Depression [71–74]. In addition to assessing for psychiatric comorbidities, chronic pruritus also negatively impairs sleep as well as quality of life (QOL). Tools to measure sleep impairment include the Athens Insomnia Scale, Stanford Sleepiness Scale, Pittsburgh Sleep Quality Index, and Epworth Sleepiness Scale [75–78].

Tools to assess quality of life commonly include the ItchyQoL, 36-item short form (SF-36) and Dermatological Life Quality Index (DLQI) [79–81]. The ItchyQoL questionnaire is specific to pruritic symptoms effects on the quality of life and is comprised of 22 items. Its questions cover symptoms, function, patients' emotions and self-perception in regard to their pruritus. The SF-36 focuses on similar aspects such as limitations and emotional impairment but is also used for conditions other than chronic pruritus [81]. Lastly, the DLQI is a validated questionnaire asking about the impact of a patient's dermatological disease and its treatment on the quality of life [80].

7. Discussion

Prurigo nodularis is an orphan disease with no standardized diagnostic or treatment regimen and has been understudied compared to other inflammatory skin diseases. Given the highly pruritic and chronic nature of this disease, there is a very high burden of disease, including high rates of associated anxiety and depression among PN patients [82]. These quality of life issues are compounded by the poor management of patients and lack of effective therapies. Greater attention is needed to formulate standardized diagnostic algorithms in the evaluation of PN patients. In particular, from our systematic review, we would like to highlight the need for a targeted clinical examination and laboratory evaluation to exclude other diagnoses and associated etiologic factors.

More randomized controlled studies with large patient cohorts are needed for uncovering more targeted treatments. As several agents are in the pipeline, greater recognition of PN and an evidence-based diagnostic workup is necessary for optimal patient management.

8. Conclusions

PN is a chronic inflammatory skin disease that often has an immense psychosocial impact on patients' quality of life. Due to its varying clinical presentations and several mimickers, we propose a diagnostic workup for those with clinically-suspected PN. More consistent diagnoses of PN could improve future studies on PN and help discover more effective therapies for patients.

Author Contributions: The following contributions were made by the authors: conceptualization: C.D.K., R.K., K.A.W., M.M.K., and S.G.K.; methodology: C.D.K., R.K., K.A.W., M.M.K., and S.G.K.; writing—original draft preparation: C.D.K.; writing—review and editing: C.D.K. and S.G.K.; visualization: C.D.K. and S.G.K.; supervision: S.G.K.

Funding: This research received no external funding.

Conflicts of Interest: Shawn G. Kwatra is an advisory board member for Menlo and Trevi Therapeutics and has received grant funding from Kiniksa Pharmaceuticals. He is also the recipient of a Dermatology Foundation Medical Dermatology Career Development Award.

References

1. Boozalis, E.; Tang, O.; Patel, S.; Semenov, Y.R.; Pereira, M.P.; Ständer, S.; Kang, S.; Kwatra, S.G. Ethnic differences and comorbidities of 909 prurigo nodularis patients. *J. Am. Acad. Dermatol.* **2018**, *79*, 714–719.e3. [CrossRef] [PubMed]
2. Larson, V.A.; Tang, O.; Stander, S.; Miller, L.S.; Kang, S.; Kwatra, S.G. Association between prurigo nodularis and malignancy in middle-aged adults. *J. Am. Acad. Dermatol.* **2019**. [CrossRef]
3. Whang, K.A.; Kang, S.; Kwatra, S.G. Inpatient Burden of Prurigo Nodularis in the United States. *Medicines* **2019**, *6*, 88. [CrossRef] [PubMed]
4. Huang, A.H.; Canner, J.K.; Khanna, R.; Kang, S.; Kwatra, S.G. Real-world prevalence of prurigo nodularis and burden of associated diseases. *J. Investig. Dermatol.* **2019**. [CrossRef] [PubMed]
5. Iking, A.; Grundmann, S.; Chatzigeorgakidis, E.; Phan, N.Q.; Klein, D.; Ständer, S. Prurigo as a symptom of atopic and non-atopic diseases: Aetiological survey in a consecutive cohort of 108 patients. *J. Eur. Acad. Dermatol. Venereol.* **2013**, *27*, 550–557. [CrossRef] [PubMed]
6. Zeidler, C.; Yosipovitch, G.; Ständer, S. Prurigo Nodularis and Its Management. *Dermatol. Clin.* **2018**, *36*, 189–197. [CrossRef]
7. Schedel, F.; Schürmann, C.; Metze, D.; Ständer, S. [Prurigo. Clinical definition and classification]. *Hautarzt* **2014**, *65*, 684–690. [CrossRef]
8. Al-Salhi, W.; Alharithy, R. Pemphigoid nodularis. *J. Cutan. Med. Surg.* **2015**, *19*, 153–155. [CrossRef]
9. Kwong, H.L.; Lim, S.P. Pemphigoid nodularis mimicking nodular prurigo in an immune-suppressed patient with rheumatoid arthritis. *Acta Derm. Venereol.* **2015**, *95*, 237–238. [CrossRef]
10. Ray, J.; Michael, C. Pemphigoid nodularis: Two new cases demonstrating distinguishing clinical clues from prurigo nodularis. *J. Am. Acad. Dermatol.* **2009**, *60*, AB103–AB104.
11. Ross, J.S.; McKee, P.H.; Smith, N.P.; Shimizu, H.; Griffiths, W.A.D.; Bhogal, B.S.; Black, M.M. Unusual variants of pemphigoid: From pruritus to pemphigoid nodularis. *J. Cutan. Pathol.* **1992**, *19*, 212–216. [CrossRef] [PubMed]
12. Powell, A.M.; Albert, S.; Gratian, M.J.; Bittencourt, R.; Bhogal, B.S.; Black, M.M. Pemphigoid nodularis (non-bullous): A clinicopathological study of five cases. *Br. J. Dermatol.* **2002**, *147*, 343–349. [CrossRef] [PubMed]
13. Seo, S.; Fischer, A. Actinic prurigo. *J. Am. Acad. Dermatol.* **2016**, *74*, AB224.
14. Pustover, K.; Fivenson, D. Epidermolysis bullosa acquisita: A unique clinical presentation with Blaschkoid acral distribution. *J. Am. Acad. Dermatol.* **2017**, *76*, AB124.
15. Pai, V.; Naveen, K.; Athanikar, S.; Rai, V.; Shastry, D. Epidermolysis bullosa pruriginosa: A report of two cases. *Indian Dermatol. Online J.* **2014**, *5*, 44–47. [CrossRef] [PubMed]
16. Ankad, B.S.; Beergouder, S.L. Hypertrophic lichen planus versus prurigo nodularis: A dermoscopic perspective. *Dermatol. Pract. Concept.* **2016**, *6*, 9–15. [CrossRef] [PubMed]

17. Werbel, T.; Hinds, B.R.; Cohen, P.R. Scabies presenting as cutaneous nodules or malar erythema: Reports of patients with scabies surrepticius masquerading as prurigo nodularis or systemic lupus erythematosus. *Dermatol. Online J.* **2018**.
18. Wick, M.R. Psoriasiform dermatitides: A brief review. *Semin. Diagn. Pathol.* **2017**, *34*, 220–225. [CrossRef]
19. Tan, W.S.; Tey, H.L. Extensive prurigo nodularis: Characterization and etiology. *Dermatology* **2014**, *228*, 276–280. [CrossRef]
20. Lee, S.; Wang, H.Y.; Kim, E.; Hwang, H.J.; Choi, E.; Lee, H.; Choi, E.H. Clinical characteristics and genetic variation in atopic dermatitis patients with and without allergic contact dermatitis. *Eur. J. Dermatol.* **2018**, *28*, 637–643.
21. Akarsu, S.; Ozbagcivan, O.; Ilknur, T.; Semiz, F.; Inci, B.B.; Fetil, E. Xerosis cutis and associated co-factors in women with prurigo nodularis. *An. Bras. Dermatol.* **2018**, *93*, 671–679. [CrossRef] [PubMed]
22. Miyachi, Y.; Okamoto, H.; Furukawa, F.; Imamura, S. Prurigo nodularis. A possible relationship to atopy. *J. Dermatol.* **1980**, *7*, 281–283. [CrossRef] [PubMed]
23. Roenigk, R.K.; Dahl, M.V. Bullous pemphigoid and prurigo nodularis. *J. Am. Acad. Dermatol.* **1986**, *14 Pt 2*, 944–947. [CrossRef]
24. Wu, T.P.; Miller, K.; Cohen, D.E.; Stein, J.A. Keratoacanthomas arising in association with prurigo nodules in pruritic, actinically damaged skin. *J. Am. Acad. Dermatol.* **2013**, *69*, 426–430. [CrossRef] [PubMed]
25. Rowland Payne, C.M.; Wilkinson, J.D.; McKee, P.H.; Jurecka, W.; Black, M.M. Nodular prurigo—A clinicopathological study of 46 patients. *Br. J. Dermatol.* **1985**, *113*, 431–439. [CrossRef] [PubMed]
26. Winhoven, S.; Gawkrodger, D. Nodular prurigo: Metabolic diseases are a common association. *Clin. Exp. Dermatol.* **2006**, *32*, 224–225. [CrossRef] [PubMed]
27. Matthews, S.N.; Cockerell, C.J. Prurigo nodularis in HIV-infected individuals. *Int. J. Dermatol.* **1998**, *37*, 401–409. [CrossRef]
28. Rien, B.E.; Lemont, H.; Cohen, R.S. Prurigo nodularis: As association with uremia. *J. Am. Podiatry Assoc.* **1982**, *72*, 321–323. [CrossRef]
29. Rishi, R.; Ringwala, S.; Tracy, J.; Fatteh, S. Prurigo nodularis and Hashimoto thyroiditis. *Ann. Allergy Asthma Immunol.* **2014**, *113*, 673–674. [CrossRef]
30. Dumont, S.; Péchère, M.; Toutous Trellu, L. Chronic Prurigo: An Unusual Presentation of Hodgkin Lymphoma. *Case Rep. Dermatol.* **2018**, *10*, 122–126. [CrossRef]
31. Seshadri, P.; Rajan, S.J.; George, I.A.; George, R. A sinister itch: Prurigo nodularis in Hodgkin lymphoma. *J. Assoc. Physicians India* **2009**, *57*, 715–716. [PubMed]
32. Parcheta, P.; Stepien, P.; Zarebska-Michaluk, D.; Krecisz, B. Nodular prurigo as first manifestation of primary biliary cholangitis successfully treated with rifampin and sertraline. *Acta Derm. Venereol.* **2017**, *97*, 1056.
33. Savoia, F.; Casadio, C.; Tabanelli, M.; Spadola, G.; Zago, S.; Maio, V.; Giacomoni, P.; Gaddoni, G.; Patrizi, A.; Lanzanova, G. Prurigo nodularis as the first manifestation of a chronic autoimmune cholestatic hepatitis. *Int. J. Dermatol.* **2011**, *50*, 1588–1589. [CrossRef] [PubMed]
34. Neri, S.; Raciti, C.; D'Angelo, G.; Ierna, D.; Bruno, C.M. Hyde's prurigo nodularis and chronic HCV hepatitis. *J. Hepatol.* **1998**, *28*, 161–164. [CrossRef]
35. Böhme, T.; Heitkemper, T.; Mettang, T.; Phan, N.Q.; Ständer, S. [Clinical features and prurigo nodularis in nephrogenic pruritus]. *Hautarzt* **2014**, *65*, 714–720. [CrossRef] [PubMed]
36. Kremer, A.E.; Wolf, K.; Ständer, S. [Intrahepatic cholestasis of pregnancy: Rare but important]. *Hautarzt* **2017**, *68*, 95–102. [CrossRef] [PubMed]
37. Larson, V.A.; Tang, O.; Ständer, S.; Kang, S.; Kwatra, S.G. Association between itch and cancer in 16,925 patients with pruritus: Experience at a tertiary care center. *J. Am. Acad. Dermatol.* **2019**, *80*, 931–937. [CrossRef] [PubMed]
38. Lin, J.T.; Wang, W.H.; Yen, C.C.; Yu, I.T.; Chen, P.M. Prurigo nodularis as initial presentation of metastatic transitional cell carcinoma of the bladder. *J. Urol.* **2002**, *168*, 631–632. [CrossRef]
39. Fina, L.; Grimalt, R.; Berti, E.; Caputo, R. Nodular prurigo associated with Hodgkin's disease. *Dermatologica* **1991**, *182*, 243–246. [CrossRef]
40. Stefanini, G.F.; Resta, F.; Marsigli, L.; Gaddoni, G.; Baldassarri, L.; Caprio, G.P.; Degli Azzi, I.; Foschi, F.G.; Gasbarrini, G. Prurigo nodularis (Hyde's prurigo) disclosing celiac disease. *Hepatogastroenterology* **1999**, *46*, 2281–2284.

41. McKenzie, A.W.; Stubbing, D.G.; Elvy, B.L. Prurigo nodularis and gluten enteropathy. *Br. J. Dermatol.* **1976**, *95*, 89–92. [PubMed]
42. Saporito, L.; Florena, A.M.; Colomba, C.; Pampinella, D.; Di Carlo, P. Prurigo nodularis due to Mycobacterium tuberculosis. *J. Med. Microbiol.* **2009**, *58 Pt 12*, 1649–1651. [CrossRef]
43. Gulin, S.J.; Čeović, R.; Lončarić, D.; Ilić, I.; Radman, I. Nodular prurigo associated with mycosis fungoides—Case report. *Acta Dermatovenerol. Croat.* **2015**, *23*, 203.
44. Menni, S.; Boccardi, D.; Gualandri, L.; Cainarca, M. Prurigo nodularis in a young child with a parasitic infestation with Ascaris lumbricoides. *Eur. J. Pediatr. Dermatol.* **2009**, *19*, 31–34.
45. Guarneri, C.; Lotti, J.; Fioranelli, M.; Roccia, M.G.; Lotti, T.; Guarneri, F. Possible role of *Helicobacter pylori* in diseases of dermatological interest. *J. Biol. Regul. Homeost. Agents* **2017**, *31* (Suppl. 2), 57–77. [PubMed]
46. Neri, S.; Ierna, D.; D'Amico, R.A.; Giarratano, G.; Leotta, C. *Helicobacter pylori* and prurigo nodularis. *Hepatogastroenterology* **1999**, *46*, 2269–2272. [PubMed]
47. Jacob, C.I.; Patten, S.F. Strongyloides stercoralis infection presenting as generalized prurigo nodularis and lichen simplex chronicus. *J. Am. Acad. Dermatol.* **1999**, *41 Pt 2*, 357–361. [CrossRef]
48. Mattila, J.O.; Katila, M.L.; Vornanen, M. Slowly growing mycobacteria and chronic skin disorders. *Clin. Infect. Dis.* **1996**, *23*, 1043–1048. [CrossRef]
49. Wang, L.S.; Wu, T.S.; Wang, C.C.J.; Ku, C.L.; Hsu, Y.H.; Chang, P.Y. Mycobacterium mucogenicum infection presenting with generalized follicular hyperplasia and prurigo nodularis in an immunocompetent patient. *Int. J. Antimicrob. Agents* **2017**, *50*, S97–S98.
50. De, D.; Dogra, S.; Kanwar, A.J. Prurigo nodularis in healed herpes zoster scar: An isotopic response. *J. Eur. Acad. Dermatol. Venereol.* **2007**, *21*, 711–712. [CrossRef]
51. Biswal, S.G.; Mehta, R.D. Cutaneous Adverse Reactions of Chemotherapy in Cancer Patients: A Clinicoepidemiological Study. *Indian J. Dermatol.* **2018**, *63*, 41–46. [CrossRef] [PubMed]
52. Fattore, D.; Panariello, L.; Annunziata, M.C.; Fabbrocini, G. Prurigo nodularis and pembrolizumab: A therapeutic challenge. *Eur. J. Cancer* **2019**, *110*, 8–10. [CrossRef] [PubMed]
53. Stefanini, G.F.; Resta, F.; Marsigli, L.; Gaddoni, G.; Baldassarri, L.; Caprio, G.P.; Degli Azzi, I.; Foschi, F.G.; Gasbarrini, G. Clinical classification of itch: A position paper of the International Forum for the Study of Itch. *Acta Derm. Venereol.* **2007**, *87*, 291–294.
54. Lee, H.G.; Stull, C.; Yosipovitch, G. Psychiatric disorders and pruritus. *Clin. Dermatol.* **2017**, *35*, 273–280. [CrossRef] [PubMed]
55. Radmanesh, M.; Shafiei, S. Underlying psychopathologies of psychogenic pruritic disorders. *Psychosom. Dermatol. Psychosom.* **2001**, *2*, 130–133. [CrossRef]
56. Dazzi, C.; Erma, D.; Piccinno, R.; Veraldi, S.; Caccialanza, M. Psychological factors involved in prurigo nodularis: A pilot study. *J. Dermatol. Treat.* **2011**, *22*, 211–214. [CrossRef] [PubMed]
57. Lotti, T.; Buggiani, G.; Prignano, F. Prurigo nodularis and lichen simplex chronicus. *Dermatol. Ther.* **2008**, *21*, 42–46. [CrossRef] [PubMed]
58. Brenaut, E.; Halvorsen, J.A.; Dalgard, F.J.; Lien, L.; Balieva, F.; Sampogna, F.; Linder, D.; Evers, A.W.; Jemec, G.B.; Gieler, U.; et al. The self-assessed psychological comorbidities of prurigo in European patients: A multicentre study in 13 countries. *J. Eur. Acad. Dermatol. Venereol.* **2019**, *33*, 157–162. [CrossRef]
59. Gieler, U.; Tomas-Aragones, L.; Linder, D.; Jemec, G.; Poot, F.; Szepietowski, J.; Korte, J.; Taube, K.; Lvov, A.; Consoli, S. Self-inflicted lesions in dermatology: Terminology and classification—A position paper from the European Society for Dermatology and Psychiatry (ESDaP). *Acta Derm. Venereol.* **2013**, *93*, 4–12. [CrossRef] [PubMed]
60. Hachisuka, J.; Chiang, M.C.; Ross, S.E. Itch and neuropathic itch. *Pain* **2018**, *159*, 603–609. [CrossRef] [PubMed]
61. Misery, L.; Brenaut, E.; Le Garrec, R.; Abasq, C.; Genestet, S.; Marcorelles, P.; Zagnoli, F. Neuropathic pruritus. *Nat. Rev. Neurol.* **2014**, *10*, 408–416. [CrossRef] [PubMed]
62. Weigelt, N.; Metze, D.; Ständer, S. Prurigo nodularis: Systematic analysis of 58 histological criteria in 136 patients. *J. Cutan. Pathol.* **2010**, *37*, 578–586. [CrossRef] [PubMed]
63. Schuhknecht, B.; Marziniak, M.; Wissel, A.; Phan, N.; Pappai, D.; Dangelmaier, J.; Metze, D.; Ständer, S. Reduced intraepidermal nerve fibre density in lesional and nonlesional prurigo nodularis skin as a potential sign of subclinical cutaneous neuropathy. *Br. J. Dermatol.* **2011**, *165*, 85–91. [CrossRef] [PubMed]

64. Pereira, M.P.; Pogatzki-Zahn, E.; Snels, C.; Vu, T.-H.; Üçeyler, N.; Loser, K.; Sommer, C.; Evers, A.W.M.; Van Laarhoven, A.I.M.; Agelopoulos, K.; et al. There is no functional small-fibre neuropathy in prurigo nodularis despite neuroanatomical alterations. *Exp. Dermatol.* **2017**, *26*, 969–971. [CrossRef] [PubMed]
65. Pereira, M.P.; Ständer, S. Assessment of severity and burden of pruritus. *Allergol. Int.* **2017**, *66*, 3–7. [CrossRef] [PubMed]
66. Reich, A.; Heisig, M.; Phan, N.; Taneda, K.; Takamori, K.; Takeuchi, S.; Furue, M.; Blome, C.; Augustin, M.; Ständer, S.; et al. Visual analogue scale: Evaluation of the instrument for the assessment of pruritus. *Acta Derm. Venereol.* **2012**, *92*, 497–501. [CrossRef]
67. Phan, N.; Blome, C.; Fritz, F.; Gerss, J.; Reich, A.; Ebata, T.; Augustin, M.; Szepietowski, J.; Ständer, S. Assessment of pruritus intensity: Prospective study on validity and reliability of the visual analogue scale, numerical rating scale and verbal rating scale in 471 patients with chronic pruritus. *Acta Derm. Venereol.* **2012**, *92*, 502–507. [CrossRef]
68. Majeski, C.J.; Johnson, J.A.; Davison, S.N.; Lauzon, C.J. Itch Severity Scale: A self-report instrument for the measurement of pruritus severity. *Br. J. Dermatol.* **2007**, *156*, 667–673. [CrossRef] [PubMed]
69. Pölking, J.; Zeidler, C.; Schedel, F.; Osada, N.; Augustin, M.; Metze, D.; Pereira, M.P.; Yosipovitch, G.; Bernhard, J.D.; Ständer, S. Prurigo Activity Score (PAS): Validity and reliability of a new instrument to monitor chronic prurigo. *J. Eur. Acad. Dermatol. Venereol.* **2018**, *32*, 1754–1760. [CrossRef]
70. Ständer, S.; Zeidler, C.; Riepe, C.; Steinke, S.; Fritz, F.; Bruland, P.; Soto-Rey, I.; Storck, M.; Agner, T.; Augustin, M.; et al. European EADV network on assessment of severity and burden of Pruritus (PruNet): First meeting on outcome tools. *J. Eur. Acad. Dermatol. Venereol.* **2016**, *30*, 1144–1147. [CrossRef]
71. Herrmann, C. International experiences with the Hospital Anxiety and Depression Scale—A review of validation data and clinical results. *J. Psychosom. Res.* **1997**, *42*, 17–41. [CrossRef]
72. Snaith, R.P. The hospital anxiety and depression scale. *Br. J. Gen. Pract.* **1990**, *40*, 305. [PubMed]
73. Hamilton, M. A rating scale for depression. *J. Neurol. Neurosurg. Psychiatry* **1960**, *23*, 56–62. [CrossRef] [PubMed]
74. Beck, A.T.; Guth, D.; Steer, R.A.; Ball, R. Screening for major depression disorders in medical inpatients with the Beck Depression Inventory for Primary Care. *Behav. Res. Ther.* **1997**, *35*, 785–791. [CrossRef]
75. Soldatos, C.R.; Dikeos, D.G.; Paparrigopoulos, T.J. Athens Insomnia Scale: Validation of an instrument based on ICD-10 criteria. *J. Psychosom. Res.* **2000**, *48*, 555–560. [CrossRef]
76. Doneh, B. Epworth Sleepiness Scale. *Occup. Med. (Lond.)* **2015**, *65*, 508. [CrossRef] [PubMed]
77. Lee, K.A.; Hicks, G.; Nino-Murcia, G. Validity and reliability of a scale to assess fatigue. *Psychiatry Res.* **1991**, *36*, 291–298. [CrossRef]
78. MacLean, A.W.; Fekken, G.C.; Saskin, P.; Knowles, J.B. Psychometric evaluation of the Stanford Sleepiness Scale. *J. Sleep Res.* **1992**, *1*, 35–39. [CrossRef]
79. Desai, N.S.; Poindexter, G.B.; Monthrope, Y.M.; Bendeck, S.E.; Swerlick, R.A.; Chen, S.C. A pilot quality-of-life instrument for pruritus. *J. Am. Acad. Dermatol.* **2008**, *59*, 234–244. [CrossRef]
80. Twiss, J.; Meads, D.M.; Preston, E.P.; Crawford, S.R.; McKenna, S.P. Can we rely on the Dermatology Life Quality Index as a measure of the impact of psoriasis or atopic dermatitis? *J. Investig. Dermatol.* **2012**, *132*, 76–84. [CrossRef]
81. Ware, J.E.; Sherbourne, C.D. The MOS 36-item short-form health survey (SF-36). I. Conceptual framework and item selection. *Med. Care* **1992**, *30*, 473–483. [CrossRef] [PubMed]
82. Jørgensen, K.M.; Egeberg, A.; Gislason, G.H.; Skov, L.; Thyssen, J.P. Anxiety, depression and suicide in patients with prurigo nodularis. *J. Eur. Acad. Dermatol. Venereol.* **2017**, *31*, e106–e107. [CrossRef] [PubMed]

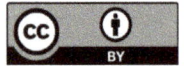

© 2019 by the authors. Licensee MDPI, Basel, Switzerland. This article is an open access article distributed under the terms and conditions of the Creative Commons Attribution (CC BY) license (http://creativecommons.org/licenses/by/4.0/).

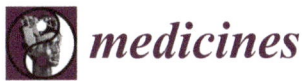

Article

Inpatient Burden of Prurigo Nodularis in the United States

Katherine A. Whang [1], Sewon Kang [1] and Shawn G. Kwatra [1,2,*]

[1] Department of Dermatology, Johns Hopkins University School of Medicine, Baltimore, MD 21205, USA
[2] Department Bloomberg School of Public Health, Johns Hopkins Bloomberg School of Public Health, Baltimore, MD 21205, USA
* Correspondence: skwatra1@jhmi.edu; Tel.: +1-410-955-8662

Received: 29 June 2019; Accepted: 8 August 2019; Published: 11 August 2019

Abstract: Background: Although prurigo nodularis (PN) has a significant burden of disease, little is known about its epidemiology and disease burden within the United States. We describe the characteristics of hospitalized patients diagnosed with PN and assess the factors associated with hospitalization. **Methods:** We performed a cross-sectional study of the 2016 National Inpatient Sample, a representative sample of 20% of hospital discharges nationally. **Results:** Patients diagnosed with PN accounted for 3.7 inpatient visits per 100,000 discharges nationally in 2016. Patients with PN were more likely to be black (odds ratio (OR) 4.43, 95% CI (3.33–6.08), $p < 0.001$) or Asian (OR 3.44, 95% CI (1.39–5.08), $p = 0.003$) compared with white patients. Patients diagnosed with PN had both a longer length of hospital stay (mean ± SD, 6.51 ± 0.37 days vs. 4.62 ± 0.02 days, $p < 0.001$) and higher cost of care ($14,772 ± $964 vs. $11,728 ± $106, $p < 0.001$) compared with patients without PN. Patients with PN were significantly more likely to be admitted for HIV complications (OR 78.2, 95% CI (46.4–131.8), $p < 0.001$). PN contributes to increased inpatient cost of care and length of hospitalization. **Conclusions:** There are racial disparities associated with hospital admission of patients diagnosed with PN.

Keywords: prurigo nodularis; pruritus; itch; inpatient; disease burden; national inpatient sample

1. Introduction

Prurigo nodularis (PN) is a chronic pruritic condition that is characterized by repeated scratching behavior and the presence of multiple, intensely itchy nodules [1]. These lesions often are excoriated to the point of ulceration and are symmetrically distributed on the extensor surfaces of the limbs and trunk [2]. PN has a significant impact on the quality of life and is linked with numerous systemic and psychological comorbidities, such as anxiety, depression, and sleep disturbance, as has been found with other pruritic conditions, like atopic dermatitis [3–7]. Recent studies on the pathogenetic mechanisms of PN has revealed the importance of pro-inflammatory cytokines, such as IL-31, and neuropeptides in lesional skin that may contribute to altered nerve density and increased inflammation in PN [8–10]. Despite the tremendous burden of disease of PN, there is very little known about the etiology and epidemiology of PN. A German study examined 108 PN patients in a predominantly Caucasian population and observed a female predominance (64%) with a median age of 61.5 years and found that more than half of PN cases had an atopic predisposition or concomitant atopic dermatitis [2]. In fact, Tanaka et al describe two distinct forms of PN: An early-onset atopic form and a late-onset non-atopic form [11]. Our group also recently described a cohort of PN patients seen in the Johns Hopkins Health System, though epidemiologic conclusions are difficult to draw based on a single health system experience [5,12].

One potential reason for the limited amount of epidemiologic data available is that PN is fairly uncommon, and in the past was grouped together with other chronic pruritic conditions in previous disease classification systems [1]. However, in 2015, the United States transitioned to the new disease classification system, International Classification of Diseases, Tenth Revision, Clinical Modification (ICD-10-CM), from the previously used ICD-9-CM, allowing for increased specificity in disease coding. For the first time, PN received a dedicated diagnosis code, enabling new avenues for epidemiologic research on PN to be explored.

Previous studies have demonstrated an association between PN and several comorbidities, such as HIV infection, hepatitis, congestive heart failure, chronic kidney disease, Type 2 diabetes mellitus, and several psychiatric conditions [5]. These conditions contribute to PN's burden of disease and may affect hospitalization and cost of care. Due to the limited research on PN as a disease entity, little is known on the inpatient burden of PN in the United States. In the current study, we analyze the epidemiology and inpatient burden of PN in the United States, as well as factors associated with hospitalization for PN in a nationally representative database of hospitalizations in 2016.

2. Materials and Methods

2.1. Data Source

We analyzed data from the National Inpatient Sample (NIS) from 2016. The NIS is administered by the Healthcare Cost and Utilization Project (HCUP) of the Agency for Healthcare Research and Quality. Each year of data represented a stratified sample of approximately 20% of all inpatient hospitalizations within the United States. Of note, 2016 was the first complete year that prurigo nodularis received an independent diagnostic code as detailed below. Sample weights provided by NIS were used to account for sampling design of hospitals to determine nationally representative estimates. The study was exempt from the institutional review board because the database was deidentified before use.

2.2. Selection of Prurigo Nodularis Cohort

Patients with a diagnosis of prurigo nodularis were selected using ICD-10-CM codes. An ICD-10-CM code of L28.1 corresponded to a diagnosis of prurigo nodularis.

2.3. Statistical Analysis

Data analysis was performed using survey models that accounted for NIS-provided survey weights, sampling clusters, and strata using Stata version 15 (StataCorp, College Station, TX, USA). We determined the estimated prevalence of hospitalization for PN. Cost of inpatient care was determined based on the total reported charge of hospitalization and the all-payer inpatient cost-to-charge ratio estimates for hospitals provided by HCUP.

The control group included all discharges with no diagnosis of PN, representing the population of hospitalized patients in the United States. In order to determine risk factors for hospitalization of patients diagnosed with PN, binary logistic models were constructed using hospitalization with PN as the dependent variable. Independent variables included age, gender, race/ethnicity, the median annual income of the hospital ZIP code, health insurance type, season of admission, hospital location, teaching status, and hospital bed capacity. A p-value of <0.05 was considered significant with Bonferroni correction.

3. Results

There was a total of 7,135,090 discharges reported in the NIS dataset during 2016. There were 265 hospitalized patients with a diagnosis of PN (weighted 1325, 95% confidence interval (CI) (1120–1530)) or 3.7 inpatient visits per 100,000 discharges in 2016.

3.1. Factors Associated with Hospitalization for Prurigo Nodularis

Patients admitted as inpatients to hospitals with a diagnosis of PN were on average older than patients without a diagnosis of PN (mean ± SD 55.2 ± 0.9 years vs. 49.0 ± 0.2 years, respectively).

Patients with PN were more likely to be black (survey-weighted logistic regression; odds ratio (OR) 4.43, 95% CI (3.33–6.08), $p < 0.001$), Hispanic (OR 1.77, 95% CI (1.09–2.88), $p = 0.02$), or Asian (OR 3.44, 95% CI (1.39–5.08), $p = 0.003$) compared with white patients (Figure 1). Black PN patients were more likely to be male than black patients of the general patient population (59.1% vs. 41.1%; OR 1.97, 95% CI (1.36–2.85), $p = 0.0003$). PN patients were also more likely to have Medicare (OR 2.81, 95% CI (1.80–4.39), $p < 0.001$) or Medicaid (OR 2.24, 95% CI (1.44–3.47), $p < 0.001$), as compared to patients with private insurance. In the US, Medicare and Medicaid are government-run programs that provide health insurance to the elderly and low-income. Hospitalized patients with PN were more likely to be seen in teaching hospitals (OR 2.60, 95% CI (1.76–3.84), $p < 0.001$) compared to non-teaching and hospitals with a large bed capacity (OR 2.15, 95% CI (1.41–3.27), $p < 0.001$).

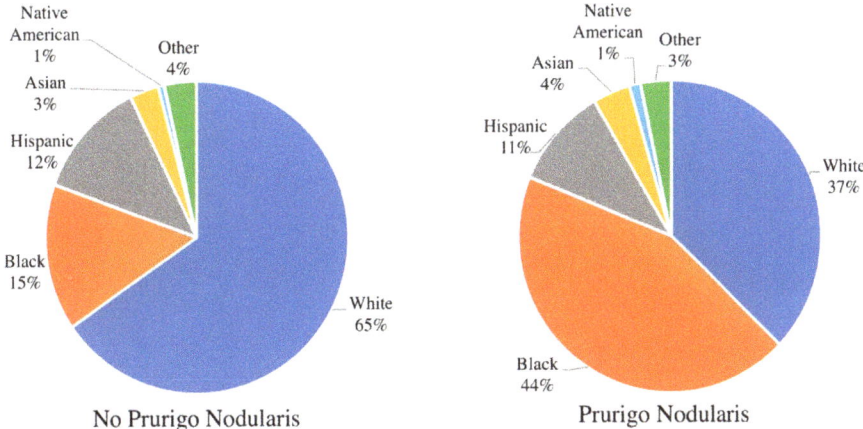

Figure 1. Comparison of racial distribution. The racial distribution of patients with no prurigo nodularis (**left**) compared to patients with prurigo nodularis (**right**). The population of prurigo nodularis patients is disproportionately black compared to patients with no prurigo nodularis.

In multivariate logistic regression models with stepwise elimination, age, race/ethnicity, insurance status, teaching status, and hospital bed size were found to have a statistically significant contribution to hospitalization for PN (Table 1). The factors of sex, income quartile, season, and hospital region were found to have no statistically significant contribution to hospitalization for PN.

Table 1. Demographics of hospitalized patients with a diagnosis of prurigo nodularis compared to the general inpatient population without a diagnosis of prurigo nodularis.

Variable	General Inpatient Population without a Diagnosis of Prurigo Nodularis		Patients with Prurigo Nodularis		Adjusted OR	p-Value
	Est. Frequency	Percent (95% Confidence Interval)	Est. Frequency	Percent (95% Confidence Interval)		
AGE, y						
0–17	5,479,694	15.3 [14.9–15.9]	5	0.38 [0.05–2.64]	0.04	0.002
18–39	7,423,759	20.8 [20.5–21.0]	210	15.8 [11.8–20.9]	1.00	—
40–59	7,403,610	20.7 [20.5–21.0]	620	46.8 [40.2–53.5]	2.95	<0.001
60–79	10,515,272	29.4 [29.0–29.7]	390	29.4 [24.0–35.5]	1.34	0.263
>80	4,886,856	13.7 [13.5–13.9]	100	7.55 [4.83–11.60]	0.75	0.386
RACE						
White	22,141,260	65.4 [64.4–66.3]	464	37.2 [30.8–44.1]	1.00	—
Black	5,145,981	15.2 [14.6–15.8]	550	44.0 [37.1–51.1]	4.43	<0.001
Hispanic	4,150,991	12.3 [11.6–12.9]	130	10.4 [6.9–15.4]	1.77	0.02
Asian	1,037,020	3.06 [2.83–3.32]	50	4.00 [2.22–7.09]	2.66	0.003
Native American	219,690	0.65 [0.56–0.75]	15	1.20 [0.39–3.67]	3.44	0.036
Other	1,156,259	3.42 [3.12–3.74]	40	3.20 [1.63–6.20]	1.29	0.586
GENDER						
Female	15,439,345	43.3 [43.1–43.5]	635	47.9 [41.7–54.2]	1.00	—
Male	20,236,076	56.7 [56.5–56.9]	690	52.1 [45.8–58.3]	1.00	0.75
SEASON						
Winter	8,914,808	25.0 [25.0–25.0]	400	30.2 [24.9–36.1]	1.00	—
Spring	9,015,068	25.3 [25.2–25.3]	315	23.8 [19.3–29.0]	0.81	0.213
Summer	8,914,118	25.0 [25.0–25.0]	305	23.0 [18.2–28.7]	0.73	0.106
Fall	8,796,723	24.7 [24.6–24.7]	270	20.4 [15.9–25.8]	0.72	0.063

Table 1. *Cont.*

Variable	General Inpatient Population without a Diagnosis of Prurigo Nodularis		Patients with Prurigo Nodularis		Adjusted OR	p-Value
	Est. Frequency	Percent (95% Confidence Interval)	Est. Frequency	Percent (95% Confidence Interval)		
INCOME QUARTILE						
First	10,774,519	30.7 [29.8–31.6]	465	36.9 [30.4–43.9]	1.00	—
Second	8,915,683	25.4 [24.8–26.0]	270	21.4 [16.5–27.3]	0.98	0.929
Third	8,387,702	23.9 [23.4–24.5]	290	23.0 [17.9–29.1]	1.18	0.398
Fourth	6,999,502	20.0 [19.0–20.9]	235	18.7 [13.2–24.0]	1.38	0.112
INSURANCE						
Medicare	14,127,590	39.6 [39.1–40.1]	645	49.0 [42.8–55.4]	2.81	<0.001
Medicaid	8,241,094	23.1 [22.6–23.7]	370	28.1 [22.7–34.3]	2.24	<0.001
Private	10,734,828	30.1 [29.6–30.6]	205	15.6 [11.6–20.7]	1.00	—
Self-pay	1,377,983	3.87 [3.71–4.03]	65	4.94 [2.84–8.48]	1.61	0.238
No charge	111,960	0.31 [0.27–0.37]	0			—
Other	1,058,214	2.97 [2.77–3.19]	30	2.28 [1.03–4.96]	1.28	0.612
INSURED						
Yes	33,078,581	92.7 [92.5–92.9]	1,220	92.1 [88.0–94.9]	1.00	—
No	1,377,983	3.86 [3.70–4.03]	65	4.91 [2.81–8.42]	1.00	—
Other or no charge	1,170,174	3.28 [3.07–3.50]	30	2.26 [1.03–4.92]	1.00	—
REGION						
Northeast	6,599,084	18.5 [17.9–19.2]	270	20.4 [15.3–26.6]	1.00	—
Midwest	7,933,647	22.2 [21.6–22.9]	355	26.8 [20.2–34.6]	1.38	0.14
South	14,041,126	39.3 [38.5–40.1]	445	33.6 [26.6–41.3]	0.91	0.649
West	7,122,759	20.0 [19.4–20.6]	255	19.2 [14.0–25.9]	1.25	0.328

Table 1. Cont.

Variable	General Inpatient Population without a Diagnosis of Prurigo Nodularis		Patients with Prurigo Nodularis		Adjusted OR	p-Value
	Est. Frequency	Percent (95% Confidence Interval)	Est. Frequency	Percent (95% Confidence Interval)		
TEACHING STATUS						
Nonteaching	23,291,422	65.4 [64.7–66.1]	1,130	85.3 [79.9–89.4]	1.00	—
Teaching	12,320,949	34.6 [33.9–35.3]	195	14.7 [10.6–20.1]	2.60	<0.001
HOSPITAL BED CAPACITY						
Small	6,674,756	18.7 [18.1–19.3]	170	12.8 [9.1–17.7]	1.00	—
Medium	10,351,226	29.0 [28.4–29.7]	240	18.1 [13.3–24.2]	1.13	0.629
Large	18,632,207	52.2 [51.5–53.0]	915	69.1 [62.1–75.2]	2.15	<0.001

3.2. Length of Stay and Cost of Care

The length of stay (LOS) in the hospital was longer in duration for patients with a diagnosis of PN compared with patients without PN (mean ± SD, 6.51 ± 0.37 days vs. 4.62 ± 0.02 days, $p < 0.001$). In multivariate linear regression for LOS in patients diagnosed with PN, older age (≥18 years) was associated with a longer duration of hospital stay (beta coefficient = 3.46, 95% CI [0.93–5.99], $p = 0.007$) (Table 2).

Table 2. Multivariate linear regression for the cost of care and length of stay among prurigo nodularis patients.

Demographic	Cost of Care			Length of Stay		
	Adjusted Beta	95% CI	p-Value	Adjusted Beta	95% CI	p-Value
AGE, y						
0–17	Reference					
18–39	8980.12	[2271.54–15688.7]	0.009	3.46	[0.93–5.99]	0.007
40–59	10306.25	[3295.591–17316.91]	0.004	2.72	[0.20–5.24]	0.034
60–79	17129.11	[8512.382–25745.83]	<0.001	3.74	[0.99–6.50]	0.008
>80	7701.64	[−1590.12–16993.42]	0.104	1.06	[−2.43–4.57]	0.55
SEASON						
Winter	Reference					
Spring	2428.98	[−3651.91–8509.88]	0.433	0.34	[−2.05–2.74]	0.776
Summer	−2276.29	[−6883.1–2330.51]	0.333	−2.08	[−4.08–−0.08]	0.041
Fall	−1365.68	[−6400.697–3669.33]	0.595	−2.06	[−4.28–0.15]	0.069
GENDER						
Female	Reference					
Male	−2927.89	[−7155.95–1300.16]	0.175	−0.23	[−1.84–1.38]	0.781
RACE						
White	Reference					
Black	−696.01	[−5725.16–4333.13]	0.786	0.18	[−2.06–2.42]	0.875
Hispanic	2806.11	[−4865.536–10477.76]	0.473	−0.28	[−2.97–2.42]	0.841
Asian	5474.29	[−1684.91–12633.5]	0.134	−0.38	[−3.27–2.50]	0.794
Native American	5100.59	[−9957.69–20158.88]	0.507	4.44	[−3.10–11.99]	0.248
Other	−6695.23	[−14271.62–881.14]	0.083	−2.55	[−5.51–0.41]	0.092
INCOME QUARTILE						
First	Reference					
Second	1357.71	[−4561.79–7277.22]	0.653	1.47	[−1.26–4.20]	0.29
Third	−326.29	[−4849.39–4196.79]	0.888	0.25	[−1.59–2.09]	0.793
Fourth	2211.26	[−5600.19–10022.73]	0.579	−0.41	[−2.73–1.90]	0.725
INSURANCE						
Medicare	3799.07	[−2029.32–9627.46]	0.201	2.14	[−0.31–4.59]	0.87
Medicaid	4274.12	[−666.47–9214.72]	0.09	2.14	[−0.07–4.35]	0.058
Private	Reference					
Self-pay	−200.49	[−6367.36–5966.37]	0.949	0.23	[−2.88–3.32]	0.886
No charge						
Other	355.35	[−8232.30–8943.01]	0.935	3.37	[−0.96–7.70]	0.127

Table 2. Cont.

Demographic	Cost of Care			Length of Stay		
	Adjusted Beta	95% CI	p-Value	Adjusted Beta	95% CI	p-Value
REGION						
Northeast	Reference					
Midwest	1947.42	[−5246.55–9141.39]	0.596	−0.84	[−3.76–2.08]	0.573
South	951.9	[−4984.18–6888.00]	0.753	0.12	[−2.44–2.68]	0.929
West	2914.19	[−4681.94–10510.34]	0.452	−0.48	[−3.35–2.40]	0.745
TEACHING STATUS						
Nonteaching	Reference					
Teaching	1639.64	[−2697.30–5976.59]	0.459	−0.22	[−2.15–1.70]	0.819
HOSPITAL BED CAPACITY						
Small	Reference					
Medium	5096.48	[−1453.24–11646.2]	0.127	0.51	[−2.35–3.37]	0.727
Large	7446.41	[1527.81–13365.01]	0.014	0.6	[−1.57–2.77]	0.587

The total cost of care for hospitalized patients diagnosed with PN was $18,686,522 in 2016; however, the actual total cost was higher because 12 patients had missing values for cost. The average cost of care was higher in patients diagnosed with PN compared with patients without PN ($14,772 ± $964 vs. $11,728 ± $106, $p < 0.001$). In multivariate linear regression for cost of care in patients diagnosed with PN, older age (≥18 years) was associated with increased cost (age under 18 years: Beta coefficient = $8,980, 95% CI (2,271.54–15,688.7), $p = 0.009$) (Table 2).

3.3. Primary Reason for Admission of Prurigo Nodularis Patients

The most common reasons for admission to the hospital for patients diagnosed with PN were sepsis (11.7%), cellulitis (7.9%), acute exacerbation of congestive heart failure (7.5%), HIV (5.7%), pneumonia (3.4%), and end stage renal disease (3.0%) (Figure 2). Patients with PN were significantly more likely to be admitted due to HIV complications compared to the general inpatient population (OR 78.2, 95% CI (46.4–131.8), $p < 0.001$). Furthermore, PN patients with concomitant HIV were significantly more likely to be black than white (OR 8.2, 95% CI (1.02–66.0), $p = 0.048$).

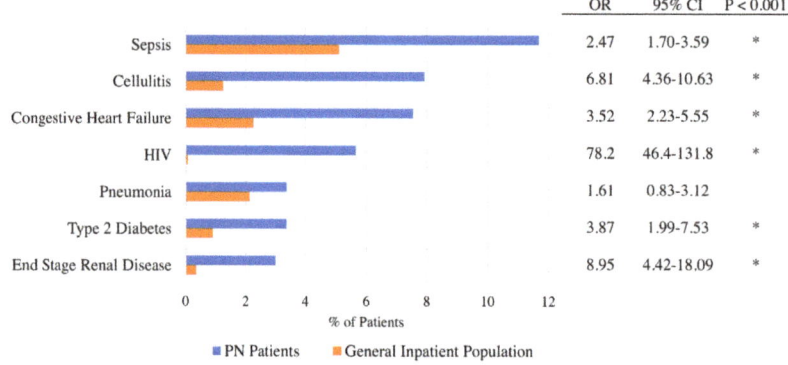

Figure 2. Comparison of primary admission reason. Primary admission reason for prurigo nodularis patients compared to patients with no prurigo nodularis.

4. Discussion

This study represents the first epidemiological investigation of PN employing a national dataset in the United States to be reported in the literature. We estimate that approximately 1325 patients diagnosed with PN were hospitalized in the United States in 2016 or 3.7 inpatients per 100,000 discharges. These PN patients had both longer hospital stays and increased costs of care as compared to the general inpatient population. This is likely to be an underestimation of the overall PN inpatient burden as there is a lack of disease awareness among most physicians, and many patients do not receive inpatient dermatology consultations. We demonstrate that PN patients are more likely than the general population to be older in age, particularly in the 40 to 59 years age range and that increased age was associated with longer hospital stay and increased the cost of care. We attribute these age-related differences to the increased concomitant systemic comorbidities with age, such as diabetes mellitus and chronic kidney disease, which are systemic causes themselves of chronic pruritus and have been found to be associated with PN [5].

Our study also demonstrates increased rates of hospitalization in PN patients who were non-white, demonstrating racial disparities in the presentation of PN. In particular, these results confirmed recent findings indicating that PN disproportionately affected blacks [5]. Indeed, among the different races studied, blacks had the greatest likelihood of having PN. As previously described, black PN patients were also more likely than whites, Asians, or Hispanics to have concomitant HIV infection [5]. We found that black patients with a PN diagnosis were significantly more likely to be male compared to the general population of black patients. Recent findings have demonstrated that out of all new HIV diagnoses to black individuals in 2017, 76% were male, which may explain the increased likelihood of black males with PN [13].

Interestingly, infections including cellulitis and sepsis were frequent reasons for admission among patients with PN. Excoriation of skin nodules to the point of ulceration may serve as a nidus for infection in PN patients. In addition, given that PN is reported to have a positive predictive value for a CD4 count of <200 among HIV patients [14], PN patients are also likely to be at greater risk of infection because of more frequent rates of immunosuppression. Increased frequency of end stage renal disease and congestive heart failure as reasons for admission are also consistent with prior studies showing an association between cardiovascular and renal comorbidities in patients with PN [5,15,16].

Strengths of this study include the use of a nationally representative dataset with over 7 million records. Given the recent transition from ICD-9-CM to ICD-10-CM, this is the first study that provides epidemiologic data on PN in the United States. Weaknesses include the small PN sample size given the under-recognition of PN by non-dermatologic specialties. Effects of disease severity and treatment on hospitalization could also not be determined.

In conclusion, our study characterizes the inpatient burden of PN in the United States and demonstrates increased cost and length of hospital stay in the care of these patients. Our study also confirms racial differences in the burden of PN, with PN patients most likely to be black. PN patients were also found to be more likely to be admitted for infections and comorbid cardiovascular and renal conditions. Additional studies are needed to further characterize the ambulatory disease burden of PN.

Author Contributions: Conceptualization, K.A.W., S.K. and S.G.K.; data curation, K.A.W. and S.G.K.; formal analysis, K.A.W.; funding acquisition, S.G.K.; investigation, K.A.W. and S.G.K.; methodology, K.A.W. and S.G.K.; supervision, S.K. and S.G.K.; validation, K.A.W.; writing—original draft, K.A.W. and S.G.K.; writing—review and editing, K.A.W., S.K. and S.G.K.

Funding: This research received no external funding.

Institutional Review Board Status: IRB approval was waived as only anonymous aggregate level data were used.

Acknowledgments: Kwatra received a research grant from the Skin of Color Society and is a recipient of a Medical Dermatology Career Development Award from the Dermatology Foundation.

Conflicts of Interest: S.G.K. is an advisory board member for Menlo and Trevi Therapeutics and has received grant funding from Kiniksa Pharmaceuticals. S.K. is an advisory board member for Menlo Therapeutics.

References

1. Pereira, M.P.; Steinke, S.; Zeidler, C.; Forner, C.; Riepe, C.; Augustin, M.; Bobko, S.; Dalgard, F.; Elberling, J.; Garcovich, S.; et al. European academy of dermatology and venereology European prurigo project: Expert consensus on the definition, classification and terminology of chronic prurigo. *J. Eur. Acad. Dermatol. Venereol.* **2018**, *32*, 1059–1065. [CrossRef] [PubMed]
2. Klein, D.; Phan, N.Q.; Grundmann, S.; Chatzigeorgakidis, E.; Iking, A.; Ständer, S. Prurigo as a symptom of atopic and non-atopic diseases: Aetiological survey in a consecutive cohort of 108 patients. *J. Eur. Acad. Dermatol. Venereol.* **2012**, *27*, 550–557.
3. Konda, D.; Chandrashekar, L.; Rajappa, M.; Kattimani, S.; Thappa, D.M.; Ananthanarayanan, P.H. Serotonin and interleukin-6: Association with pruritus severity, sleep quality and depression severity in Prurigo Nodularis. *Asian J. Psychiatry* **2015**, *17*, 24–28. [CrossRef] [PubMed]
4. Schneider, G.; Driesch, G.; Heuft, G.; Evers, S.; Luger, T.A.; Ständer, S. Psychosomatic cofactors and psychiatric comorbidity in patients with chronic itch. *Clin. Exp. Dermatol.* **2006**, *31*, 762–767. [CrossRef] [PubMed]
5. Boozalis, E.; Tang, O.; Patel, S.; Semenov, Y.R.; Pereira, M.P.; Stander, S.; Kang, S.; Kwatra, S.G. Ethnic differences and comorbidities of 909 prurigo nodularis patients. *J. Am. Acad. Dermatol.* **2018**, *79*, 714–719. [CrossRef] [PubMed]
6. Boccardi, D.; D'Auria, E.; Turati, F.; DI Vito, M.; Sortino, S.; Riva, E.; Cerri, A. Disease severity and quality of life in children with atopic dermatitis: PO-SCORAD in clinical practice. *Minerva Pediatr.* **2017**, *69*, 373–380. [PubMed]
7. Coutanceau, C.; Stalder, J. Analysis of Correlations between Patient-Oriented SCORAD (PO-SCORAD) and Other Assessment Scores of Atopic Dermatitis Severity. *Dermatology* **2014**, *229*, 248–255. [CrossRef] [PubMed]
8. Kneiber, D.; Valdebran, M.; Amber, K.T. Treatment-resistant prurigo nodularis: Challenges and solutions. *Clin. Cosmet. Investig. Dermatol.* **2019**, *12*, 163–172.
9. Sonkoly, E.; Muller, A.; Lauerma, A.I.; Alenius, H.; Dieu-nosjean, M.; Meller, S.; Ruzicka, T.; Zlotnik, A.; Homey, B. IL-31: A new link between T cells and pruritus in atopic skin inflammation. *J. Allergy Clin. Immunol.* **2006**, *117*, 411–417. [CrossRef] [PubMed]
10. D'Auria, E.; Banderali, G.; Barberi, S.; Gualandri, L.; Pietra, B. Atopic dermatitis: Recent insight on pathogenesis and novel therapeutic target. *Asian Pac. J. Allergy Immunol.* **2016**, *34*, 98–108.
11. Tanaka, M.; Aiba, S.; Matsumura, N.; Aoyama, H.; Tagami, H. Prurigo nodularis consists of two distinct forms: Early-onset atopic and late-onset non-atopic. *Dermatology* **1995**, *190*, 269–276. [CrossRef]
12. Larson, V.A.; Tang, O.; Stander, S.; Miller, L.S.; Kang, S.; Kwatra, S.G. Association between prurigo nodularis and malignancy in middle-aged adults. *J. Am. Acad. Dermatol.* **2019**. [CrossRef] [PubMed]
13. Diagnoses of HIV Infection in the United States and Dependent Areas. 2017. Available online: http://www.cdc.gov/hiv/library/reports/hiv-surveillance.html (accessed on 2 August 2019).
14. Magand, F.; Nacher, M.; Cazorla, C.; Cambazard, F.; Marie, D.S.; Couppié, P. Predictive values of prurigo nodularis and herpes zoster for HIV infection and immunosuppression requiring HAART in French Guiana. *Trans. R. Soc. Trop. Med. Hyg.* **2011**, *105*, 401–404. [CrossRef] [PubMed]
15. Yang, M.; Tang, W.; Sang, Y.; Chen, X.; Hu, X. Prevalence of chronic kidney disease-associated pruritus among adult dialysis patients. *Medicine* **2018**, *97*, 10633.
16. Winhoven, S.M.; Gawkrodger, D.J. Nodular prurigo: Metabolic diseases are a common association. *Clin. Exp. Dermatol.* **2007**, *32*, 224–225. [CrossRef] [PubMed]

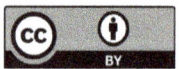

© 2019 by the authors. Licensee MDPI, Basel, Switzerland. This article is an open access article distributed under the terms and conditions of the Creative Commons Attribution (CC BY) license (http://creativecommons.org/licenses/by/4.0/).

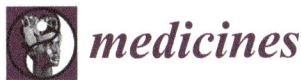

Article

Association between Prurigo Nodularis and Etiologies of Peripheral Neuropathy: Suggesting a Role for Neural Dysregulation in Pathogenesis

John-Douglas Matthew Hughes [1,*], Taylor E. Woo [2], Micah Belzberg [3], Raveena Khanna [3], Kyle A. Williams [3], Madan M. Kwatra [4], Shahzeb Hassan [5] and Shawn G. Kwatra [3]

1. Department of Medicine, Division of Dermatology, University of Calgary, Calgary, AB T2T 5C7, Canada
2. Cumming School of Medicine, University of Calgary, Calgary, AB T2N 4N1, Canada; tewoo@ucalgary.ca
3. Department of Dermatology, Johns Hopkins University School of Medicine, Baltimore, MD 21205, USA; mbelzbe@jhu.edu (M.B.); rkhanna8@jhmi.edu (R.K.); kwill184@health.fau.edu (K.A.W.); skwatra1@jhmi.edu (S.G.K.)
4. Department of Anesthesiology, Duke University Medical Center, Durham, NC 27710, USA; madan.kwatra@duke.edu
5. Feinberg School of Medicine, Northwestern University, Chicago, IL 60611, USA; shahzeb.hassan@northwestern.edu
* Correspondence: john.hughes@ucalgary.ca

Received: 14 October 2019; Accepted: 26 December 2019; Published: 8 January 2020

Abstract: Background: Prurigo nodularis (PN) is an intensely pruritic skin condition of considerable morbidity. However, the pathogenesis of PN and its association with underlying neuropathy is unclear. **Objective**: We sought to investigate the association between PN and etiologies of peripheral neuropathy. **Methods**: A cross-sectional analysis of adult patients (≥18-year-old) with PN, AD, and Psoriasis at the Johns Hopkins Health System over a six-year period (January 2013–January 2019) was performed. The strength of association with etiologies of peripheral neuropathy were compared to a control cohort of individuals without PN, as well as those with AD or psoriasis. **Results**: A total of 1122 patients with PN were compared to 10,390 AD patients, 15,056 patients with psoriasis, and a control cohort of 4,949,017 individuals without PN, with respect to 25 comorbidities associated with peripheral neuropathies. **Limitations**: Comparisons between peripheral neuropathies and PN represent associations but are not causal relationships. **Conclusion**: Prurigo nodularis is strongly associated with peripheral neuropathies, suggesting a role for neural dysregulation in pathogenesis.

Keywords: prurigo nodularis; nodular prurigo; pruritus; itch; neuropathy

1. Introduction

Prurigo nodularis (PN) is a chronic skin condition characterized by intensely pruritic nodules and hyperkeratotic lesions. Lesions are distributed symmetrically with involvement of extensor surfaces of the extremities. The intractable pruritus of PN is a significant contributor of morbidity for patients and commonly presents in the context of known pruritic conditions [1]. It is associated with other dermatologic conditions, such as atopic dermatitis and other systemic diseases [2]. Examples of systemic diseases associated with PN include liver or kidney dysfunction, hyperthyroidism, metabolic dysfunction, inflammatory processes, psychological factors, and malignancy [3–5]. The underlying mechanism of how these conditions contribute to the pathogenesis of PN remains unclear; however, neural dysregulation is thought to play a central role.

Recent studies have studied intraepidermal nerve fiber density (IENFD) as an important contributor to chronic pruritus and in small fiber neuropathies [6,7]. Patients with PN are observed to have decreased IENFD as compared to healthy individuals [7]. Furthermore, there is a significant reduction in IENFD in lesional PN skin, which may be due to prolonged scratching, but also in non-lesional PN [5]. Indeed, the resolution of pruritus is associated with the recovery of dermal nerve fiber density [6]. Cellular changes observed in patients with PN include increased concentrations of substance P and calcitonin gene-related peptide (CGRP) in the nerve fibers of PN patients [8]. Whether these neurophysiological changes are markers of an underlying neuropathies or are a result of the intractable pruritus remains controversial [9]. However, treatments commonly used to treat neuropathic pain have been shown to benefit PN. Agents such as gabapentin and pregabalin have been successfully used to treat patients with PN [10–12]. Thalidomide has also been successfully used to treat refractory cases of prurigo nodularis [13,14].

With the evidence surrounding a neural origin of PN unclear, we sought to understand the association between PN and peripheral neuropathies. Furthermore, we conducted a cross-sectional investigation in our health system, comparing patients with PN to individuals with psoriasis, and those with atopic dermatitis.

2. Materials and Methods

An association between PN and peripheral neuropathies was investigated by using the Johns Hopkins Health System (JHHS) electronic medical record system, EPIC. The JHHS is a representative collection of approximately 25–30 million individuals located in a 200-mile area within Maryland and its neighboring states and is inclusive of individuals traveling from other countries to the JHHS. Institutional review board approval was not required, as only anonymous, aggregate-level data were used.

A cross-sectional study was performed of patients aged 18 years and older seen at JHHS between 1 January 2013 and 1 January 2019 (n = 4,950,139). EPIC Slicer Dicer was used to collect anonymized aggregate-level data; consequently, IRB approval was waived. SNOMED CT search terms were applied to separately identify patients with PN, atopic dermatitis (AD), psoriasis, or patients without PN. Disease-specific search terms were then applied to identify the prevalence of patients within each group diagnosed with each selected peripheral-neuropathy-related condition. Odds ratios were calculated by comparing the prevalence of patients with PN and each comorbidity to the prevalence of patients in each group with the same comorbidity. Then, p-values were calculated, using chi-squared tests with one degree of freedom. To account for multiple comparisons, a Bonferroni-corrected p-value was applied. Associations were considered statistically significant if $p < 0.05$.

3. Results

3.1. Patient Demographics

A total of 1122 adult patients with PN, 10,390 AD patients, and 15,056 patients with psoriasis were identified over the six-year period (Figure 1). A control cohort consisting of 4,949,017 individuals without PN was used. In the general population, there was a predominance of Caucasians (61.3%), with African American individuals only representing 21.3% of the patients within the JHHS. Similarly, Caucasians represented over 76.6% of the psoriasis group. In comparison, PN and AD cohorts had differing representative populations. The PN cohort was composed of 41.9% Caucasian and 47.6% African American individuals. Similarly, the AD cohort had 43% and 40.5% of Caucasian and African American patients, respectively.

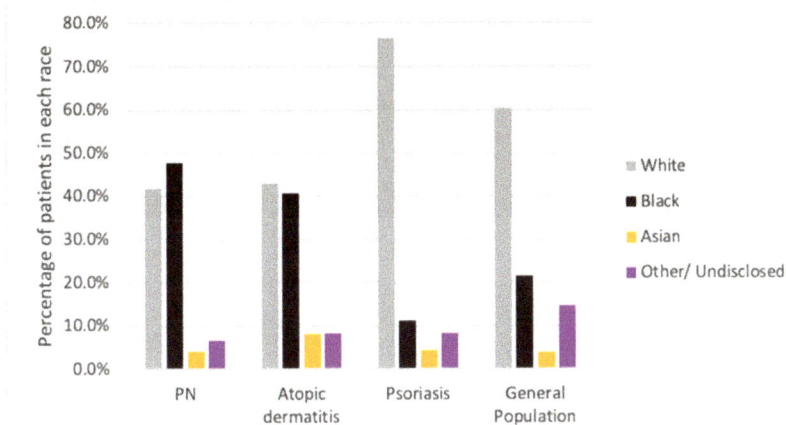

Figure 1. Racial backgrounds of all patients 18 years and older with a diagnosis of prurigo nodularis (PN), atopic dermatitis (AD), or psoriasis, and within the general population who presented to the Johns Hopkins Hospital System between 1 January 2013 and 1 January 2019.

Within the PN study cohort, the proportion of males and females was similar as compared to the general population, with 52% females and 48% males within the PN cohort, and 54.2% females and 45.5% males within the general population. The mean age of PN patients was 56, similar to the general population (56) and the psoriasis cohort (55) (Figure 2). Individuals with atopic dermatitis were comparatively younger, with a mean age of 45. The prevalence of PN increased with age, with the peak prevalence seen between 50 and 59 years of age and composing 26.5% of our cohort. A total of 67.4% of all patients with PN were between 40 and 69 years of age, with individuals between the years of 50 and 59 composing 26.5% of the cohort.

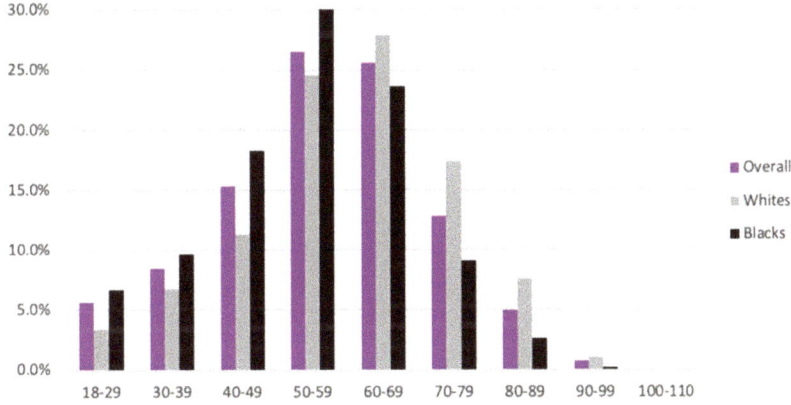

Figure 2. Age distribution of patients with prurigo nodularis (PN) overall, in black and in white patients.

3.2. Association of Prurigo Nodularis with Conditions Known to Feature Peripheral Neuropathies

Individuals with PN were more likely to have comorbidities associated with peripheral neuropathies as compared to the general population (Table 1). The most common comorbidities seen in patients with PN were statin use (37.34%), diabetes mellitus (26.38%), chronic kidney disease (16.04%), human influenza virus (HIV, 13.37%), metronidazole use (12.39%), and hypothyroidism (11.05%). All the comorbidities analyzed were significantly more common in the PN group, with the exception of small-cell carcinoma ($p = 0.09$). Of the significant comorbidities, borreliosis (Lyme disease) was weakly associated with PN (OR: 3.6, IQR 1.5–8.6, $p < 0.00001$). In contrast, patients with PN were 58 times more likely to have HIV as compared to the general population (OR: 58, IQR 48.8–68.9, $p < 0.00001$). External agents associated with comorbidities of peripheral neuropathies include the use of dapsone, alcohol use, statins, and metronidazole ($p < 0.00001$). Both cobalamin deficiency and folic acid deficiency were associated with peripheral neuropathies in patients with PN. Lastly, inflammatory processes, chronic kidney disease, and neoplasms were associated strongly with PN, including vasculitis ($p < 0.000001$), chronic kidney disease (OR 16.3; 95% CI 13.9–19.2; $p < 0.00001$), and primary malignant neoplasms ($p < 0.00001$). Other conditions, including diabetes mellitus, hyperpituitarism, hypothyroidism, and the presence of myxedema, carpal tunnel syndrome, ulnar nerve entrapment, amyloidosis, vasculitis, and phlebitis, were associated with PN.

We next examined whether significant differences existed between patients with PN, atopic dermatitis, and psoriasis (Table 1). Among the many differences, patients with PN were more likely to have chronic kidney disease and HIV as compared to both comparator groups ($p < 000001$). However, there were no differences with malignant processes and metabolic conditions, including hyperpituitarism and primary malignant neoplasms, such as small-cell carcinoma and non-small-cell carcinoma. In comparison to atopic dermatitis, no significant differences were observed between carpal tunnel syndrome, use of metronidazole, folic acid deficiency, or hypothyroidism. When comparing the PN cohort to the psoriasis cohort, patients with PN were more likely to have comorbidities associated with peripheral neuropathies, with the exception of myxedema, borreliosis, PMN, folic acid deficiency, and Waldenstrom's macroglobulinemia.

Table 1. Absolute number, percentage, odds ratios, and *p*-values of all patients 18 years and older with PN and various comorbid conditions, as compared with those of patients 18 and older with AD, with psoriasis, or within the general population (without PN) who were seen at the JHHS between 1 January 2013 and 1 January 2019.

Comorbidity	PN, n (%)	AD, n (%)	OR (95% CI)	*p*-Value	Psoriasis, n (%)	OR (95% CI)	*p*-Value	Gen Pop, n (%)	OR (95% CI)	*p*-Value
Peripheral neuropathies	308(27.45)	1673(16.1)	1.97(1.71–2.27)	<0.002	2759(18.32)	1.69(1.47–1.94)	<0.002	150,325(3.04)	12.08(10.59–13.77)	<0.002
Focal–multifocal neuropathies										
Amyloidosis	12(1.07)	31(0.3)	3.61(1.85–7.05)	<0.002	32(0.21)	5.08(2.61–9.88)	<0.002	2234(0.05)	23.94(13.53–42.35)	<0.002
Carpal tunnel syndrome	54(4.81)	397(3.82)	1.27(0.95–1.7)	0.10377	522(3.47)	1.41(1.06–1.88)	0.01893	22,079(0.45)	11.28(8.58–14.83)	<0.002
DM	296(26.38)	1167(11.23)	2.83(2.45–3.28)	<0.002	2648(17.59)	1.68(1.46–1.93)	<0.002	177,323(3.58)	9.64(8.44–11.01)	<0.002
Hyperpituitarism	6(0.53)	37(0.36)	1.5(0.63–3.57)	0.35138	38(0.25)	2.12(0.9–5.04)	0.07978	3268(0.07)	8.14(3.64–18.16)	<0.002
Myxedema	5(0.45)	15(0.14)	3.1(1.12–8.53)	0.02133	27(0.18)	2.49(0.96–6.48)	0.05277	1169(0.02)	18.95(7.86–45.69)	<0.002
Phlebitis	26(2.32)	122(1.17)	2(1.3–3.06)	<0.002	168(1.12)	2.1(1.38–3.19)	<0.002	7395(0.15)	15.85(10.74–23.4)	<0.002
Ulnar nerve entrapment	17(1.52)	74(0.71)	2.14(1.26–3.65)	0.00391	76(0.5)	3.03(1.79–5.15)	<0.002	3546(0.07)	21.46(13.27–34.68)	<0.002
Vasculitis	38(3.39)	208(2)	1.72(1.21–2.44)	0.00231	302(2.01)	1.71(1.22–2.41)	<0.002	13,241(0.27)	13.07(9.45–18.07)	<0.002
Chronic axonal neuropathies										
Alcohol abuse	69(6.15)	202(1.94)	3.3(2.5–4.38)	<0.002	462(3.07)	2.07(1.6–2.69)	<0.002	33,073(0.67)	9.74(7.63–12.43)	<0.002
Borreliosis	5(0.45)	63(0.61)	0.73(0.29–1.83)	0.50450	141(0.94)	0.47(0.19–1.16)	0.09351	62,20(0.13)	3.56(1.48–8.57)	0.00250
CKD	180(16.04)	446(4.29)	4.26(3.54–5.13)	<0.002	950(6.31)	2.84(2.39–3.37)	<0.002	57,268(1.16)	16.32(13.91–19.15)	<0.002
Cobalamin deficiency	31(2.76)	204(1.96)	1.42(0.97–2.08)	0.07200	383(2.54)	1.09(0.75–1.58)	0.65366	13,782(0.28)	10.17(7.12–14.55)	<0.002
Dapsone	48(4.28)	132(1.27)	3.47(2.48–4.86)	<0.002	96(0.64)	6.97(4.9–9.9)	<0.002	5420(0.11)	40.76(30.49–54.5)	<0.002
Folic acid deficiency	5(0.45)	14(0.13)	3.32(1.19–9.23)	0.01480	30(0.2)	2.24(0.87–5.79)	0.08659	930(0.02)	23.82(9.87–57.47)	<0.002
HIV infection	150(13.37)	185(1.78)	8.51(6.8–10.66)	<0.002	144(0.96)	15.98(12.6–20.27)	<0.002	13,137(0.27)	57.98(48.78–68.92)	<0.002
Hypothyroidism	124(11.05)	844(8.12)	1.41(1.15–1.72)	<0.002	2066(13.72)	0.778(0.64–0.95)	0.01169	113,182(2.29)	5.31(4.4–6.4)	<0.002
Metronidazole	139(12.39)	1216(11.7)	1.07(0.88–1.29)	0.49875	1098(7.29)	1.8(1.49–2.17)	<0.002	69,631(1.41)	9.91(8.3–11.84)	<0.002
NSCLC	3(0.27)	9(0.09)	3.09(0.84–11.44)	0.07466	33(0.22)	1.22(0.37–3.99)	0.74091	2234(0.05)	5.94(1.91–18.45)	<0.002
Phenytoin	2(0.18)	1(0.01)	18.55(1.68–204.76)	<0.002	2(0.01)	13.44(1.89–95.52)	<0.002	1039(0.02)	8.5(2.12–34.09)	<0.002
PMN	94(8.38)	432(4.16)	2.11(1.67–2.66)	<0.002	894(5.94)	1.45(1.16–1.81)	<0.002	73,237(1.48)	6.09(4.93–7.52)	<0.002
PMN of Lung	6(0.53)	30(0.29)	1.86(0.77–4.47)	0.16086	83(0.55)	0.97(0.42–2.23)	0.94261	7227(0.15)	3.68(1.65–8.2)	<0.002
PMN of Ovary	2(0.18)	4(0.04)	4.64(0.85–25.34)	0.05135	4(0.03)	6.72(1.23–36.73)	0.01090	481(0.01)	18.37(4.58–73.76)	<0.002

Table 1. Cont.

Comorbidity	PN, n (%)	AD, n (%)	OR (95% CI)	p-Value	Psoriasis, n (%)	OR (95% CI)	p-Value	Gen Pop, n (%)	OR (95% CI)	p-Value
Small-cell carcinoma	1(0.09)	4(0.04)	2.32(0.26–20.74)	0.43939	14(0.09)	0.96(0.13–7.3)	0.96736	948(0.02)	4.66(0.65–33.12)	0.09051
Statins	419(37.34)	1999(19.24)	2.5(2.2–2.85)	<0.002	4748(31.54)	1.29(1.14–1.47)	<0.002	361,855(7.31)	7.56(6.69–8.53)	<0.002
Waldenstrom's disease	1(0.09)	3(0.03)	3.09(0.32–29.72)	0.30358	5(0.03)	2.69(0.31–23.01)	0.34799	293(0.01)	15.07(2.11–107.42)	<0.002

Data are for all patients aged 18 years or older, including 1122 patients with prurigo nodularis (PN), 10,390 patients with AD, 15,056 patients with psoriasis, and 4,949,017 patients in the general population (excluding those with PN). PMN; primary malignant neoplasm; JHHS, Johns Hopkins Health System; CKD, chronic kidney disease; NSCLC, non-small-cell lung cancer; n/a, not applicable; OR, odds ratio; 95% CI, 95% confidence interval.

4. Discussion

The etiology of PN is complex, with both local and systemic disease contributing to the intense pruritus characteristic of the disease [15]. While underlying dermatological conditions, systemic disease, and mood disturbances have been previously associated with PN [16], a limited number of studies have been conducted investigating a neuropathic etiology of PN. Herein, we observed a significant association between PN and comorbidities of peripheral neuropathies. Many of the comorbidities examined, including chronic kidney disease, type-2 diabetes mellitus, and HIV infections, likely contribute both through their association with pruritus and the development of peripheral neuropathies [17]. Furthermore, patients with PN were more likely to have HIV as compared to patients with AD or psoriasis and may be accounted for by the role of HIV as a contributor to severe systemic pruritus [15,18].

Notably, exogenous agents and the association of drug therapies and peripheral neuropathies were observed within our cohort. The use of statins and metronidazole were both more likely to be seen in patients with PN. Evidence suggests that pruritus has been reported in up to 16% of cases associated with statins [19]. Furthermore, both statins and dapsone have been reported in the literature, for their association with peripheral neuropathies [20,21]. Metronidazole is uncommonly associated with pruritus, though it has been associated with the development of peripheral neuropathies in patients exposed to extended high-dose treatment courses [22]. The use of low-dose metronidazole has been reported in several case reports for the management of PN [23]. Lastly, there is an association between patients with PN and depression, anxiety, and greater anxiolytic use [16]. Recent evidence comparing patients with psoriasis and PN found no differences in the psychological profile with respect to the prevalence of anxiety, depression, or somatoform disorders [24]. These findings may account for the increased likelihood of alcohol abuse seen within our PN cohort and its known association with peripheral neuropathies. More importantly, our findings further emphasize the need for increased awareness and consideration of early referral for psychodynamic intervention on behalf of these patients.

Differences existing between PN, AD, and psoriasis were observed within our study. Interestingly, these differences, although in part likely due to different pathophysiology of these conditions, may also be explained by the difference in burden caused by the pruritus. A recent study examining the burden of pruritus amongst inflammatory dermatoses found that patients with PN were significantly more bothered by evening and nighttime pruritus and reported more significant impairment in quality of life as compared to patients with psoriasis and AD, despite the association of AD and PN [25,26].

We also found that PN was significantly associated with carpal tunnel syndrome, ulnar nerve entrapment, myxedema, hyperpituitarism, amyloidosis, vasculitis, and phlebitis, all of which are novel, to the best of our knowledge, with the exception of amyloidosis [27]. Malignancy was significantly associated with the PN as compared to the general population, likely due to its contributions to pruritus. Recent studies have identified that patients with PN are more likely to have been diagnosed with a malignancy as compared to the general population [28]. However, given the limited number of patients with small-cell carcinoma, it is possible that its lack of association with PN may have represented a statistical anomaly due to limited sample size.

As a cross-sectional analysis, our comparisons are limited to establishing correlations and not causative relationships between PN and peripheral neuropathies. In addition, the temporality between peripheral neuropathies and exposure to the underlying etiology is not captured by our analysis. It is likely that the pathogenesis of PN and peripheral neuropathies is multifactorial and includes variables not accounted for in our analysis. Lastly, the data are representative of a single center and are, therefore, limited in their generalizability.

5. Conclusions

Overall, this study represents a large cross-sectional analysis of PN patients' to-date, in which an association with peripheral neuropathies is observed. This association with peripheral neuropathies may suggest the importance of neuropathic changes in the pathogenesis of PN. In addition, PN demonstrates distinct differences in comparison to AD and psoriasis, despite their roles as chronic inflammatory pruritic conditions. Clinically, our study underscores an important link between PN and peripheral neuropathies. This may highlight an increased propensity for neural dysregulation in patients with PN. As such, consideration and evaluation of peripheral neuropathies should be considered in patients with PN.

Author Contributions: The authors of this manuscript contributed in the following manner: J.-D.M.H., methodology, data curation, formal analysis, original draft preparation, writing, review, editing, and funding acquisition. T.E.W., original draft preparation and editing. M.B., data curation and visualization. R.K., visualization. K.A.W., Project administration. S.H., original draft preparation. M.M.K., editing and review. S.G.K., conceptualization, editing, and supervision. All authors have read and agreed to the published version of the manuscript.

Funding: This research was funded by the Canadian Dermatology Foundation through the Frederick Kalz Bursary.

Conflicts of Interest: The authors declare no conflict of interest.

References

1. Kwon, C.D.; Khanna, R.; Williams, K.A.; Kwatra, M.M.; Kwatra, S.G. Diagnostic Workup and Evaluation of Patients with Prurigo Nodularis. *Medicines* **2019**, *6*, 97. [CrossRef]
2. Huang, A.H.; Canner, J.K.; Khanna, R.; Kang, S.; Kwatra, S.G. Real-world prevalence of prurigo nodularis and burden of associated diseases. *J. Investig. Dermatol.* **2019**. [CrossRef]
3. Székely, H.; Pónyai, G.; Temesvári, E.; Berczi, L.; Hársing, J.; Kárpáti, S.; Herszényi, L.; Tulassay, Z.; Juhasz, M. Association of collagenous colitis with prurigo nodularis. *Eur. J. Gastroenterol. Hepatol.* **2009**, *21*, 946–951. [CrossRef] [PubMed]
4. Payne, R.; Wilkinson, J.D.; Mckee, P.H.; Jurecka, W.; Black, M.M. Nodular prurigo—A clinicopathological study of 46 patients. *Br. J. Dermatol.* **1985**, *113*, 431–439. [CrossRef] [PubMed]
5. Dazzi, C.; Erma, D.; Piccinno, R.; Veraldi, S.; Caccialanza, M. Psychological factors involved in prurigo nodularis: A pilot study. *J. Dermatolog Treat.* **2011**, *22*, 211–214. [CrossRef] [PubMed]
6. Bobko, S.; Zeidler, C.; Osada, N.; Riepe, C.; Pfleiderer, B.; Pogatzki-Zahn, E.; Lvov, A.; Ständer, S. Intraepidermal Nerve Fibre Density is Decreased in Lesional and Inter-lesional Prurigo Nodularis and Reconstitutes on Healing of Lesions. *Acta Derm. Venereol.* **2016**, *96*, 404–406. [CrossRef] [PubMed]
7. Schuhknecht, B.; Marziniak, M.; Wissel, A.; Phan, N.; Pappai, D.; Dangelmaier, J.; Metze, D.; Ständer, S. Reduced intraepidermal nerve fibre density in lesional and nonlesional prurigo nodularis skin as a potential sign of subclinical cutaneous neuropathy. *Br. J. Dermatol.* **2011**, *165*, 85–91. [CrossRef] [PubMed]
8. Vaalasti, A.; Suomalainen, H.; Rechardt, L. Calcitonin gene-related peptide immunoreactivity in prurigo nodularis: A comparative study with neurodermatitis circumscripta. *Br. J. Dermatol.* **1989**, *120*, 619–623. [CrossRef] [PubMed]
9. Pereira, M.P.; Pogatzki-Zahn, E.; Snels, C.; Vu, T.H.; Üçeyler, N.; Loser, K.; Sommer, C.; Evers, A.W.M.; Van Laarhoven, A.I.M.; Agelopoulos, K.; et al. There is no functional small-fibre neuropathy in prurigo nodularis despite neuroanatomical alterations. *Exp. Dermatol.* **2017**, *26*, 969–971. [CrossRef]
10. Bharati, A.; Wilson, N.J.E. Peripheral neuropathy associated with nodular prurigo. *Clin. Exp. Dermatol.* **2017**, *26*, 969–971. [CrossRef]
11. Mazza, M.; Guerriero, G.; Marano, G.; Janiri, L.; Bria, P.; Mazza, S. Treatment of prurigo nodularis with pregabalin. *J. Clin. Pharm Ther.* **2013**, *38*, 16–18. [CrossRef] [PubMed]
12. Huang, A.H.; Canner, J.K.; Kang, S.; Kwatra, S.G. Analysis of real-world treatment patterns in patients with prurigo nodularis. *J. Am. Acad. Dermatol.* **2019**, *82*, 34–36. [CrossRef] [PubMed]
13. Aguh, C.; Kwatra, S.G.; He, A.; Okoye, G.A. Thalidomide for the Treatment of Chronic Refractory Prurigo Nodularis. *Dermatol. Online J.* **2018**, *24*, 1–6. [CrossRef]
14. Sharma, D.; Kwatra, S.G. Thalidomide for the treatment of chronic refractory pruritus. *J. Am. Acad. Dermatol.* **2016**, *74*, 363–369. [CrossRef] [PubMed]
15. Tarikci, N.; Kocatürk, E.; Güngör, Ş.; Topal, I.O.; Can, P.Ü.; Singer, R. Pruritus in Systemic Diseases: A Review of Etiological Factors and New Treatment Modalities. *Sci. World J.* **2015**. [CrossRef] [PubMed]

16. Jørgensen, K.M.; Egeberg, A.; Gislason, G.H.; Skov, L.; Thyssen, J.P. Anxiety, depression and suicide in patients with prurigo nodularis. *J. Eur. Acad. Dermatol. Venereol.* **2017**, *31*, e106–e107. [CrossRef]
17. Boozalis, E.; Tang, O.; Patel, S.; Semenov, Y.R.; Pereira, M.P.; Stander, S.; Kang, S.; Kwatra, S.G. Ethnic differences and comorbidities of 909 prurigo nodularis patients. *J. Am. Acad. Dermatol.* **2018**, *79*, 714–719.e3. [CrossRef]
18. Matthews, S.N.; Cockerell, C.J. Prurigo nodularis in, H.I.V-infected individuals. *Int J. Dermatol.* **1998**, *37*, 401–409. [CrossRef]
19. Reich, A.; Ständer, S.; Szepietowski, J.C. Drug-induced pruritus: A review. *Acta Derm.-Venereol.* **2009**, *89*, 236–244. [CrossRef]
20. Tierney, E.F.; Thurman, D.J.; Beckles, G.L.; Cadwell, B.L. Association of statin use with peripheral neuropathy in the, U.S. population 40 years of age or older. *J. Diabetes* **2012**, *5*, 207–215. [CrossRef]
21. Waldinger, T.P.; Siegle, R.J.; Weber, W.; Voorhees, J.J. Dapsone-Induced Peripheral Neuropathy. *Arch. Dermatol.* **1984**, *120*, 356–359. [CrossRef] [PubMed]
22. Goolsby, T.A.; Jakeman, B.; Gaynes, R.P. Clinical relevance of metronidazole and peripheral neuropathy: A systematic review of the literature. *Int J. Antimicrob. Agents* **2018**, *51*, 319–325. [CrossRef] [PubMed]
23. Spring, P.; Gschwind, I.; Gilliet, M. Prurigo nodularis: Retrospective study of 13 cases managed with methotrexate. *Clin. Exp. Dermatol.* **2014**, *39*, 468–473. [CrossRef] [PubMed]
24. Schneider, G.; Hockmann, J.; Ständer, S.; Luger, T.A.; Heuft, G. Psychological factors in prurigo nodularis in comparison with psoriasis vulgaris: Results of a case-control study. *Br. J. Dermatol.* **2006**, *154*, 61–66. [CrossRef] [PubMed]
25. Steinke, S.; Zeidler, C.; Riepe, C.; Bruland, P.; Soto-Rey, I.; Storck, M.; Augustin, M.; Bobko, S.; Garcovich, S.; Legat, F.J.; et al. Humanistic burden of chronic pruritus in patients with inflammatory dermatoses: Results of the European Academy of Dermatology and Venereology Network on Assessment of Severity and Burden of Pruritus (PruNet) cross-sectional trial. *J. Am. Acad. Dermatol.* **2018**, *79*, 457–463. [CrossRef] [PubMed]
26. Iking, A.; Grundmann, S.; Chatzigeorgakidis, E.; Phan, N.Q.; Klein, D.; Ständer, S. Prurigo as a symptom of atopic and non-atopic diseases: Aetiological survey in a consecutive cohort of 108 patients. *J. Eur. Acad. Dermatol. Venereol.* **2013**, *27*, 550–557. [CrossRef]
27. Baykal, C.; Ozkaya-Bayazit, E.; Gökdemir, G.; Diz Küçükkaya, R. The combined occurrence of macular amyloidosis and prurigo nodularis. *Eur. J. Dermatol.* **2000**, *10*, 297–299. Available online: http://www.ncbi.nlm.nih.gov/pubmed/10846258 (accessed on 22 October 2018).
28. Larson, V.A.; Tang, O.; Stander, S.; Miller, L.S.; Kang, S.; Kwatra, S.G. Association between prurigo nodularis and malignancy in middle-aged adults. *J. Am. Acad. Dermatol.* **2019**, *81*, 1198–1201. [CrossRef]

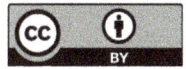

© 2020 by the authors. Licensee MDPI, Basel, Switzerland. This article is an open access article distributed under the terms and conditions of the Creative Commons Attribution (CC BY) license (http://creativecommons.org/licenses/by/4.0/).

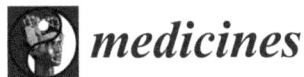

Article

Comorbidities in Mycosis Fungoides and Racial Differences in Co-Existent Lymphomatoid Papulosis: A Cross-Sectional Study of 580 Patients in an Urban Tertiary Care Center

Subuhi Kaul [1,*], Micah Belzberg [2], John-Douglas Matthew Hughes [3], Varun Mahadevan [2], Raveena Khanna [2], Pegah R. Bakhshi [2], Michael S. Hong [2], Kyle A. Williams [2], Annie L. Grossberg [2], Shawn G. Kwatra [2,†] and Ronald J. Sweren [2,†]

[1] Department of Medicine, John H. Stroger Hospital of Cook County, Chicago, IL 60612, USA
[2] Department of Dermatology, Johns Hopkins University School of Medicine, Baltimore, MD 21287, USA; mbelzbe@jhu.edu (M.B.); vmahade1@jhu.edu (V.M.); rkhanna8@jhmi.edu (R.K.); pb746@georgetown.edu (P.R.B.); michael.hong@som.umaryland.edu (M.S.H.); kwill184@health.fau.edu (K.A.W.); agrossb2@jhmi.edu (A.L.G.); skwatra1@jhmi.edu (S.G.K.); rsweren1@jhmi.edu (R.J.S.)
[3] Section of Dermatology, University of Calgary, Alberta, AB T2N 1N4, Canada; jhugh017@uottawa.ca
* Correspondence: subuhi.kaul@cookcountyhhs.org; Tel.: +1-312-864-7000
† Considered co-senior authors.

Received: 26 October 2019; Accepted: 24 December 2019; Published: 26 December 2019

Abstract: Background: Mycosis fungoides (MF) is a cutaneous T-cell lymphoma. Previous reports have suggested MF is associated with inflammatory conditions such as psoriasis, increased cardiovascular risk factors as well as secondary neoplasms. **Methods:** A cross-sectional study of MF patients seen from 2013 to 2019 was performed. Comorbidities were selected based on the 2015 Medicare report highlighting the most common chronic medical illnesses in the United States. Lifetime comorbidity occurrence in patients with MF were compared with that in patients with atopic dermatitis, psoriasis and patients without MF. Additional analyses were performed with patients sub-stratified by race. **Results:** Compared to control groups, MF was strongly associated with lymphomatoid papulosis and Hodgkin's disease, but not significantly associated with lung, breast or colon cancer. Interestingly, the association with lymphomatoid papulosis was observed in Caucasians (CI 1062-4338; $p < 0.001$) and not African Americans ($p = 0.9$). Patients with MF had a greater association with congestive heart failure, hypertension (HT) and hyperlipidemia (HLD) compared with the general population. However, they were significantly less likely to have HT and HLD when compared with psoriasis patients (HT CI: 0.6–0.9; $p < 0.001$, and HLD CI: 0.05–0.07; $p < 0.001$). MF patients were also significantly less likely to have concomitant vitamin D deficiency compared with atopic dermatitis (AD) and psoriasis ($p < 0.001$). **Conclusions:** Our results suggest that the association of MF with lymphomatoid papulosis varies by race. Compared to the general population, hypertension and hyperlipidemia were positively associated with MF, however, these were significantly less likely on comparison to psoriasis. Unlike previously described, vitamin D deficiency was found to be significantly less in patients with MF.

Keywords: mycosis fungoides; atopic dermatitis; psoriasis; associations; comorbidities; epidemiology; lymphomatoid papulosis; lymphoma; racial differences

1. Introduction

Mycosis fungoides (MF) is the most common cutaneous T-cell lymphoma (CTCL), accounting for approximately half of all primary cutaneous lymphomas [1]. Although the incidence of CTCL was rising in the 1970s, (due to either a real increase in cases, improvement in diagnostic methods, or a combination of the two) it has since stabilized to 5.6 per million persons with MF in the United States [2–4].

While most commonly observed after the age of 55 years, MF onset can arise in early adulthood or childhood with a nearly 2:1 male to female ratio [2]. MF typically has a slow and progressive disease course with patches, plaques and tumors developing sequentially. However, nearly 30% of patients demonstrate erythroderma or skin tumors at the outset [2]. Advanced disease involving blood, lymph nodes and visceral organs occurs in close to a third of cases [1]. Moreover, patients with MF are reported to be at an increased risk of developing secondary neoplasms, particularly Hodgkin lymphoma and lymphomatoid papulosis [2].

Recent evidence points to a relationship with inflammatory disorders like psoriasis—attributable to similarities in pathogenesis and the possible role of Toll-like receptors in both [5,6]. Patients with MF experience increased rates of cardiovascular risk factors [7], and apart from those experiencing limited plaque/patch stage (T1) MF, lower overall survival when compared to healthy controls matched for race, age and sex [8,9]. Being a chronic relapsing disease, the presence of comorbid conditions can potentially add to patient burden.

Considering these new observations, further investigation to elucidate the comorbidities and risk of selected malignancies associated with MF is important. To help identify the common illnesses associated with MF, a cross sectional study was conducted to evaluate 580 adult patients with diagnosed MF.

2. Materials and Methods

We performed a cross-sectional study of patients age 18 and older treated at Johns Hopkins Hospital System (JHHS) between January 1, 2013 and January 1, 2019. Johns Hopkins is a tertiary care referral center with a diverse catchment area which includes local, regional, national and international patients. Anonymous aggregate-level data was collected therefore institutional review board approval was waved. Lifetime incidences of comorbidities were collected using the electronic medical records system EPIC [10–12].

Patients diagnosed with MF were compared with three groups: all adults who presented to JHHS with diagnoses other than MF (labelled "general population" for the purpose of this study), adult patients with a diagnosis of atopic dermatitis (AD) and adults diagnosed with psoriasis. The list of comorbidities was obtained from the 2015 Medicare report of the most common chronic medical illnesses affecting the United States population [13]. Malignancies previously reported or suspected to be associated with MF such as Hodgkin's disease, malignant melanoma and cancers of the lung, breast or colon, were also included for analysis.

Odds ratios, p-values and 95% confidence intervals were calculated using chi-squared statistics with one degree of freedom. p-values for comparisons of odds ratios were calculated with Z-tests. A Bonferroni-corrected p-value of <0.001 was applied to all assessments of statistical significance. Additionally, subgroup analyses stratified by race were performed for the aforementioned comorbidities and malignancies.

3. Results

Of the 4,944,449 patients that presented to JHHS in the past six years, 580 were diagnosed with MF. Of these, 56.1% were Caucasian, 32.4% were African American and 2.9% were Asian. (Figure 1) Overall, the majority (45.1%) of the MF patients were between the ages of 60 to 79 years. However, the African American MF patients were, on average, younger than the Caucasian group—47.9% of the

African Americans belonged to the 50 to 69-year group while 50.1% of Caucasians belonged to the 60 to 79-year group (Figure 2).

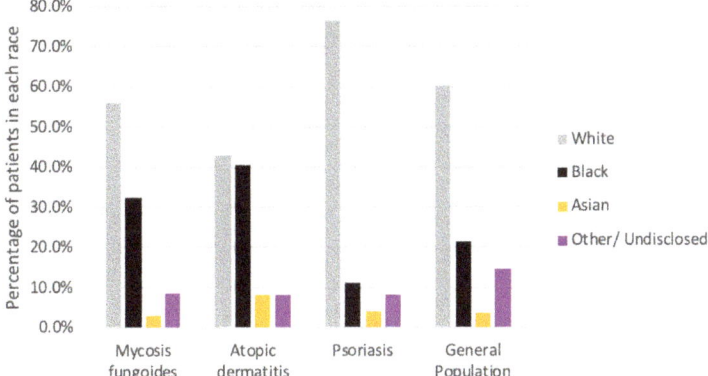

Figure 1. Racial backgrounds of all patients 18 years and older with a diagnosis of mycosis fungoides (MF), atopic dermatitis (AD), or psoriasis and within the general population who presented to the Johns Hopkins Hospital System between January 1, 2013 and January 1, 2019.

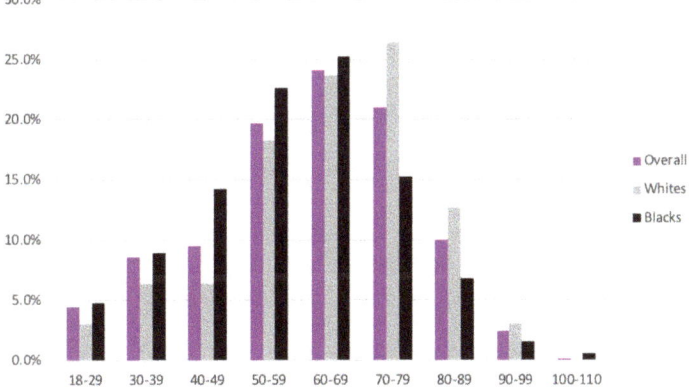

Figure 2. Age distribution of patients with mycosis fungoides (MF) overall, in black and in patients.

Overall (inclusive of all races), MF was statistically significantly associated with certain cutaneous and systemic conditions when compared with all three groups—the general population, patients with AD and patients diagnosed with psoriasis. These included major depressive disorder, Hodgkin's disease, lymphomatoid papulosis ($p < 0.001$ vs. all control groups). Patients with MF were also significantly less likely to have vitamin D deficiency ($p < 0.001$ vs. all control groups) (Table A1).

However, on stratifying by race there were important differences in the associated comorbidities. Among the Caucasian study group there was a statistically significant association with lymphomatoid papulosis ($p < 0.001$ vs. all control groups). However, no instances of lymphomatoid papulosis were observed among African American patients with MF. Additionally, on racial sub stratification the association with some conditions was lost; these included congestive heart failure and atopic dermatitis (Tables A2 and A3).

Compared with psoriasis, MF was not associated with chronic obstructive pulmonary disease (COPD), ischemic heart disease, atrial fibrillation, allergic contact dermatitis, venous thrombosis, chronic kidney disease, malignant melanoma or Alzheimer's disease. Compared with AD, MF was not associated with osteoarthritis, rheumatoid arthritis, hyperlipidemia, diabetes mellitus type 2 and psoriasis. There was no association found with chronic hepatitis C, inflammatory bowel disease, HIV, Autistic disorder, schizophrenia, ischemic stroke and lung, breast or colon cancer on comparison with AD, psoriasis and/or the general population. The number of Asian patients in our MF cohort was too small to determine associated conditions (Tables A2 and A3).

4. Discussion

This study is among the few analyses of dermatoses, malignancies and comorbidities associated with MF. In line with the literature, the majority (64.8%) of our study group were aged between 50 and 79 years [2,3]. However, in contrast to previous studies the number of females in our MF cohort outnumbered the males (51% vs. 49%) [2,3,14–16]. Concordant with earlier observations, we found that Caucasians were most commonly affected, constituting 56.1% of our patient cohort [2,8,17]. However, African Americans were disproportionately affected as compared to the general population; about 32.4% of the patients diagnosed with MF in our study were African American, whereas only 21.3% of all patients seen at JHHS over the same six-year period were African American (Figure 1). Indeed, some earlier studies have found higher incidence rates of MF in African Americans than Caucasians [3,18,19]. Our African American cohort also tended to be younger than the Caucasian group (Figure 2). These are similar to the observations of Huang et al. and are important since African Americans with MF have been found to have significantly shorter overall survival when compared with age at onset-, stage- and treatment-matched Caucasian patients [17,20].

Our study found that MF in Caucasian patients is statistically significantly associated with lymphomatoid papulosis, a finding that was not seen in our African American cohort. White patients with MF were 2147.0 times more likely to have lymphomatoid papulosis than Caucasians in the general population (odds ratio (OR) 2147.0; 95% CI 1062.6–4338.1) and 47.5 times more likely to have lymphomatoid papulosis than race-matched atopic dermatitis patients (OR 47.5; 95% CI 13.0–173.3) (Tables A2 and A3). Although, the association of MF with lymphomatoid papulosis is well known, this racial difference is significant [21]. In both our African American as well as our Caucasian study groups, MF disease was found to be statistically significantly associated with Hodgkin's disease. This confirms reports of previous studies that found an association between MF and neoplastic disorders like lymphomatoid papulosis and Hodgkin's disease [22–26]. The possible reasons for an increased risk of developing second malignancies in MF patients could either be due to the treatment used or similar dysfunctional immune surveillance leading to clonal proliferation [24,27,28]. Alternatively, the two neoplasms may have common genetic events and originator cells contributing to the development of different clones [26]. Considering the high odds of lymphomatoid papulosis and Hodgkin's disease being associated with MF, long term monitoring of MF patients is prudent regardless of the treatment protocol used. However, the significant racial difference observed suggest monitoring for development of MF may be more beneficial in Caucasian compared to African American patients with lymphomatoid papulosis.

Whether atopic dermatitis contributes to the development of MF has remained controversial. Results from previous studies have indicated a modest increase in the risk of lymphoma in patients with AD [11]. We found that overall (inclusive of all races), patients with MF were not significantly more likely to have AD when compared with patients with psoriasis ($p = 0.022$). Moreover, this was corroborated when racial sub-group analysis was performed. One possible explanation for the observations in earlier studies is early misclassification of some MF cases as AD. Due to similarities in clinical presentation, there can be a delay from the date of presentation to the diagnosis of MF. A recent study observed higher rates of pruritus associated with malignancies, particularly in case of cutaneous lymphoma in blacks which may add to the difficulty in initial diagnosis [29]. Also, often long term or treatment refractory cases labelled AD may get re-biopsied and demonstrate MF.

A recent retrospective analysis demonstrated that about 12.7% (41 of 321) of the MF patients had associated psoriasis; of these, 20 patients had psoriasis coexistent with MF. The authors of this study suggested that this association was less likely due to misclassification and could be due to the underlying abnormal T-cell activation in psoriasis which can potentially contribute to the development of cancer [5]. However, contrary to their observations, we found that when compared with patients with AD, MF patients were not significantly more likely to have psoriasis (OR 1.1; CI 0.7–1.7; $p = 0.6$), suggesting that misclassification contributes to an inflated number of psoriasis cases thought to be associated with MF. Nevertheless, further investigation into this may be warranted.

Vitamin D deficiency has earlier been thought to play a role in triggering MF [30]. In contrast, our study found that MF patients (all races) were 4.6 times ($p < 0.001$) significantly less likely to have vitamin D deficiency than the general population. This is maintained on subgroup analysis: Caucasian MF patients were significantly less likely to have concomitant vitamin D deficiency compared with AD, psoriasis and general population ($p < 0.001$). Our African American cohort was also significantly less likely to have vitamin D deficiency when compared with the general population (Table A2). These observations diverge from that of Talpur et al. who found about 77% of their CTCL patients to be deficient in vitamin D deficiency [31]. One rationale could be the use of phototherapy which may have led to improved vitamin D levels in our cohort, however, further longitudinal studies may be required for confirmation.

Interestingly, our data identified a statistically significant association with congestive heart failure, compared with the general population and AD. This association was maintained on sub stratification by race—both Caucasian and African American patients had a significant association with congestive heart failure. Also, there was a significant association with important coronary artery disease (CAD) risk factors, hypertension and hyperlipidemia (OR 5.3 and 5.0, respectively; $p < 0.001$), when compared with the general population. The association was comparable on racial sub-group analysis (Tables A1–A3). A possible explanation for this could be that acquired cardiovascular diseases as well as common coronary artery disease (CAD) risk factors (hypertension and hyperlipidemia) are more frequent beyond middle age which is the most commonly affected age group in MF [32]. However, Cengiz et al. recently demonstrated an increased rate of cardiovascular risk factors (hyperlipidemia, high homocysteine and high-sensitivity C-reactive protein) in a cohort of MF patients who did not have pre-existing metabolic disease and were lifetime non-smokers, suggesting a real increase in cardiovascular morbidity by virtue of MF [7]. This begs the chicken or the egg dilemma: are these patients at risk for developing the risk factors for cardiovascular disease (CVD), or do they also have an increased risk of CVD independent of known changes in risk factors or perhaps MF exacerbates risk factors. Further examination of cardiovascular disease and CAD risk factors in MF is suggested by these findings. However, when compared with psoriasis the association of MF with important CAD risk factors, hypertension and hyperlipidemia, was significantly less likely ($p < 0.001$). This held true for all sub-group analyses except in the case of hyperlipidemia in African Americans (Tables A1–A3).

Our study has several limitations. First, its cross-sectional design prohibits determining a temporal relationship. The data was representative of the population seen at a single tertiary care hospital system in the United States and thus, may not be generalizable. Also, misclassification of early MF as morphologically similar dermatoses like atopic dermatitis, contact dermatitis and psoriasis is possible and could potentially contribute to an inflated percentage of these dermatoses showing up in our results. Additionally, the comparison group "general population" in our study refers to the total population excluding patients with MF, however, since patients with AD and psoriasis are included in this group it may lead to an overestimation or underestimation of results. Moreover, as aggregate level data was used, gender information missing at the time of analysis may account for our unexpected sex distribution. Finally, there may be additional unknown confounding factors such as socioeconomic status or preexisting medical comorbidities in the mycosis fungoides group that could have affected the interpretation of our results.

5. Conclusions

These results indicate that MF is strongly associated with Hodgkin's disease, and that MF in Caucasians is associated with lymphomatoid papulosis. This finding in this study suggests that clinicians consider long term follow up for Caucasian but not African American patients with lymphomatoid papulosis to monitor for development of MF. Moreover, we found that although MF is significantly associated with CAD risk factors compared with the general population, these associations were less likely on comparison with psoriasis. On comparison with clinical mimickers, MF was not significantly associated with contact dermatitis (compared with psoriasis) and psoriasis (compared with AD) or lung, breast and colon cancer, conditions that have previously been thought to be associated with MF.

Author Contributions: Study was conceptualized by S.K., M.B., J.-D.M.H., S.G.K. and R.J.S. Study methodology was developed with contributions by all authors (S.K., M.B., J.-D.M.H., V.M., R.K., P.R.B., M.S.H., K.A.W., A.L.G., S.G.K. and R.J.S.). Data analyses was performed by S.K., M.B., J.-D.M.H., V.M., R.K. and K.A.W. Original draft preparation, review and editing was performed by all authors (S.K., M.B., J.-D.M.H., V.M., R.K., P.R.B., M.S.H., K.A.W., A.L.G., S.G.K. and R.J.S.). Data visualization was performed by S.K., M.B. and J.-D.M.H. Software: M.S.H. Project supervision and administration was performed by S.G.K. and R.J.S. All authors have read and agreed to the published version of the manuscript.

Funding: This research received no external funding.

Conflicts of Interest: Shawn G. Kwatra is on the advisory board for Menlo and Trevi Therapeutics and has received grant funding from Kiniksa Pharmaceuticals. The other author(s) have no conflicts of interest to declare.

Appendix A

Table A1. Absolute number, percentage, odds ratios and p values of all patients 18 years and older with MF and various comorbid conditions, as compared with those of patients 18 and older with AD, with psoriasis, or within the general population (without MF) who were seen at the Johns Hopkins Hospital System (JHHS) between January 1, 2013 and January 1, 2019. Data presented for 580 patients with mycosis fungoides (MF), 10,382 patients with AD, 15,051 patients with psoriasis, and 4,943,869 patients in the general population (excluding those with MF). AD, Atopic dermatitis; COPD, chronic obstructive pulmonary disease; OR, odds ratio; PN, prurigo nodularis.

Comorbidity	MF, n (%)	AD, n (%)	OR (95% CI)	p Value	Psoriasis, n (%)	OR (95% CI)	p Value	Gen Pop, n (%)	OR (95% CI)	p Value
Allergic Contact Dermatitis	6 (1.0)	428 (4.1)	0.2 (0.1–0.5)	<0.001	137 (0.9)	1.1 (0.5–2.6)	0.75779	4876 (0.1)	10.6 (4.7–23.7)	<0.001
Alzheimer Disease	5 (0.9)	27 (0.3)	3.3 (1.3–8.7)	0.00892	105 (0.7)	1.2 (0.5–3.0)	0.64202	8882 (0.2)	4.8 (2.0–11.7)	<0.001
Asthma	38 (6.6)	2223 (21.4)	0.3 (0.2–0.4)	<0.001	1529 (10.2)	0.6 (0.4–0.9)	0.00454	109,109 (2.2)	3.1 (2.2–4.3)	<0.001
Atopic Dermatitis	23 (4.0)				369 (2.5)	1.6 (1.1–2.5)	0.02214	10,358 (0.2)	19.7 (13.0–29.9)	<0.001
Atrial Fibrillation	32 (5.5)	284 (2.7)	2.1 (1.4–3.0)	<0.001	931 (6.2)	0.9 (0.6–1.3)	0.51122	68,394 (1.4)	4.2 (2.9–5.9)	<0.001
Autistic Disorder	0 (0)	50 (0.5)	0	0.09391	19 (0.1)	0	0.39189	2371 (0.0)	0	0.59782
Breast Cancer	2 (0.3)	33 (0.3)	1.1 (0.3–4.5)	0.91079	76 (0.5)	0.7 (0.2–2.8)	0.59126	7509 (0.2)	2.3 (0.6–9.1)	0.23285
Chronic Hepatitis C	3 (0.5)	130 (1.3)	0.4 (0.1–1.3)	0.11564	214 (1.4)	0.4 (0.1–1.1)	0.06769	13,952 (0.3)	1.8 (0.6–5.7)	0.28601
Chronic Kidney Disease	41 (7.1)	446 (4.3)	1.7 (1.2–2.4)	0.00161	950 (6.3)	1.1 (0.8–1.6)	0.46281	57,386 (1.2)	6.5 (4.7–8.9)	<0.001
Colon Cancer	0 (0)	8 (0.1)	0	0.50364	27 (0.2)	0	0.3073	2561 (0.1)	0	0.5835
Congestive Heart Failure	37 (6.4)	287 (2.8)	2.4 (1.7–3.4)	<0.001	675 (4.5)	1.5 (1.0–2.0)	0.03177	43,133 (0.9)	7.7 (5.5–10.8)	<0.001
COPD	36 (6.2)	424 (4.1)	1.6 (1.1–2.2)	0.01308	961 (6.4)	1.0 (0.7–1.4)	0.86328	51,410 (1.0)	6.3 (4.5–8.8)	<0.001
Diabetes Mellitus Type 2	64 (11.0)	103 (9.7)	1.2 (0.9–1.5)	0.27746	2191 (14.6)	0.7 (0.6–0.9)	0.01782	136,538 (2.8)	4.4 (3.4–5.7)	<0.001
HIV	3 (0.5)	185 (1.8)	0.3 (0.1–0.9)	0.02243	144 (1.0)	0.5 (0.4–0.7)	0.28188	13,283 (0.3)	1.9 (0.6–6.0)	0.24755
Hodgkin's Disease	7 (1.2)	10 (0.1)	12.7 (4.8–33.4)	<0.001	20 (0.1)	9.2 (3.9–21.8)	<0.001	1631 (0.0)	37.0 (17.5–78.1)	<0.001
Hyperlipidemia	155 (26.7)	2736 (26.4)	1.0 (0.8–1.2)	0.84364	5,812 (38.6)	0.6 (0.5–0.7)	<0.001	335,534 (6.8)	5.0 (4.2–6.0)	<0.001
Hypertension	194 (33.4)	2991 (28.8)	1.2 (1.0–1.5)	0.01664	6128 (40.7)	0.7 (0.6–0.9)	<0.001	427,318 (8.6)	5.3 (4.5–6.3)	<0.001
Inflammatory Bowel Disease	5 (0.9)	94 (0.9)	1.0 (0.4–2.3)	0.91448	228 (1.5)	0.6 (0.2–1.4)	0.203	8817 (0.2)	4.9 (2.0–11.7)	<0.001
Ischemic Heart Disease	53 (9.1)	512 (4.9)	1.9 (1.4–2.6)	<0.001	1274 (8.5)	1.1 (0.8–1.5)	0.56805	79,665 (1.6)	6.1 (4.6–8.1)	<0.001
Ischemic Stroke	0 (0)	23 (0.2)	0	0.25649	37 (0.2)	0	0.23189	2715 (0.1)	0	0.5724
Lung Cancer	3 (0.5)	30 (0.3)	1.8 (0.5–5.9)	0.32876	83 (0.6)	0.9 (0.3–3.0)	0.91295	7229 (0.1)	3.6 (1.1–11.0)	0.01939
Lymphomatoid Papulosis	11 (1.9)	4 (0.0)	50.2 (15.9–158)	<0.001	-			49 (0.0)	1950.5 (1009.0–3770.4)	<0.001

Table A1. Cont.

Comorbidity	MF, n (%)	AD, n (%)	OR (95% CI)	p Value	Psoriasis, n (%)	OR (95% CI)	p Value	Gen Pop, n (%)	OR (95% CI)	p Value
Major Depressive Disorder	44 (7.6)	1340 (12.9)	0.6 (0.4–0.8)	<0.001	2091 (13.9)	0.5 (0.4–0.7)	<0.001	119,308 (2.4)	3.3 (2.4–4.5)	<0.001
Malignant Melanoma	9 (1.6)	70 (0.7)	2.3 (1.2–4.7)	0.01504	164 (1.1)	1.4 (0.7–2.8)	0.29657	7879 (0.2)	9.9 (5.1–19.1)	<0.001
Osteoarthritis	80 (13.8)	1689 (16.3)	0.8 (0.6–1.0)	0.11477	3981 (26.5)	0.4 (0.4–0.6)	<0.001	187,109 (3.8)	4.1 (3.2–5.2)	<0.001
Osteoporosis	13 (2.2)	417 (4.0)	0.5 (0.3–1.0)	0.0321	870 (5.8)	0.4 (0.2–0.7)	<0.001	44,238 (0.9)	2.5 (1.4–4.4)	<0.001
Psoriasis	23 (4.0)	369 (3.6)	1.1 (0.7–1.7)	0.60368				15,028 (0.3)	13.5 (8.9–20.6)	<0.001
Rheumatoid Arthritis	8 (1.4)	128 (1.2)	1.1 (0.5–2.3)	0.75656	493 (3.3)	0.4 (0.2–0.8)	0.01095	11,071 (0.2)	6.2 (3.1–12.5)	<0.001
Schizophrenia	2 (0.3)	73 (0.7)	0.5 (0.1–2.0)	0.30831	71 (0.5)	0.7 (0.2–3.0)	0.66003	8507 (0.2)	2.0 (0.5–8.0)	0.31551
Venous Thrombosis	26 (4.5)	268 (2.6)	1.8 (1.2–2.7)	0.00581	496 (3.3)	1.4 (0.9–2.1)	0.11836	34,113 (0.7)	6.8 (4.6–10.0)	<0.001
Vitamin D Deficiency	65 (11.2)	2052 (19.8)	0.5 (0.4–0.7)	<0.001	2996 (19.9)	0.5 (0.4–0.7)	<0.001	132,446 (2.7)	4.6 (3.5–5.9)	<0.001

Table A2. Absolute number, percentage, odds ratios and p values of Black/African American patients age 18 years and older with mycosis fungoides and various comorbid conditions, as compared with race-matched controls age 18 years and older with AD, with psoriasis, or within the general population who were seen at the JHHS between January 1, 2013 and January 1, 2019. Data presented for 190 patients with mycosis fungoides (MF), 4287 patients with AD, 1690 patients with psoriasis, and 944,278 patients in the general population (excluding those with MF). AD, Atopic dermatitis; COPD, chronic obstructive pulmonary disease; OR, odds ratio; PN, prurigo nodularis; IBS, inflammatory bowel disease.

Comorbidity	MF, n (%)	AD, n (%)	OR (95% CI)	p Value	Psoriasis, n (%)	OR (95% CI)	p Value	Gen Pop, n (%)	OR (95% CI)	p Value
Allergic Contact Dermatitis	2 (1.1)	118 (2.8)	0.4 (0.1–1.5)	0.15571	22 (1.3)	0.8 (0.2–3.5)	0.77179	893 (0.1)	11.2 (2.8–45.3)	<0.001
Alzheimer Disease	2 (1.1)	10 (0.2)	4.6 (1.0–20.9)	0.03255	11 (0.7)	1.6 (0.4–7.4)	0.52635	1742 (0.2)	5.8 (1.4–23.2)	0.00532
Asthma	13 (9.5)	1240 (28.9)	0.3 (0.2–0.4)	<0.001	266 (15.7)	0.6 (0.3–0.9)	0.02221	40,063 (4.2)	2.4 (1.4–3.8)	<0.001
Atopic Dermatitis	11 (5.8)				93 (5.5)	1.1 (0.6–2.0)	0.86989	4276 (0.5)	13.5 (7.3–24.9)	<0.001
Atrial Fibrillation	13 (6.8)	74 (1.7)	4.2 (2.3–7.7)	<0.001	75 (4.4)	1.6 (0.9–2.9)	0.13687	10,168 (1.1)	6.7 (3.8–11.9)	<0.001
Autistic Disorder		17 (0.4)	0	0.38448	6 (0.4)	0	0.41072	687 (0.1)	0	0.70994
Breast Cancer	2 (1.1)	13 (0.3)	3.5 (0.8–15.6)	0.08025	10 (0.6)	1.8 (0.4–8.2)	0.44942	1465 (0.2)	6.8 (1.7–27.6)	0.00168
Chronic Hepatitis C	2 (1.1)	95 (2.2)	0.5 (0.1–1.9)	0.28112	64 (3.8)	0.3 (0.1–1.1)	0.05218	7057 (0.7)	1.4 (0.4–5.7)	0.62517
Chronic Kidney Disease	18 (9.5)	224 (5.2)	1.9 (1.1–3.1)	0.01127	179 (10.6)	0.9 (0.5–1.5)	0.63332	20,616 (2.2)	4.7 (2.9–7.6)	<0.001
Colon Cancer		1 (0.0)	0	0.83324	2 (0.1)	0	0.63519	461 (0.0)	0	0.76064
Congestive Heart Failure	17 (8.9)	136 (3.2)	3.0 (1.8–5.1)	<0.001	115 (6.8)	1.3 (0.8–2.3)	0.2731	13,103 (1.4)	7.0 (4.2–11.5)	<0.001
COPD	13 (6.8)	195 (4.5)	1.5 (0.9–2.8)	0.14163	120 (7.1)	1.0 (0.5–1.7)	0.89518	13,161 (1.4)	5.2 (3.0–9.1)	<0.001

Table A2. Cont.

Comorbidity	MF, n (%)	AD, n (%)	OR (95% CI)	p Value	Psoriasis, n (%)	OR (95% CI)2	p Value	Gen Pop, n (%)	OR (95% CI)	p Value
Diabetes Mellitus Type 2	34 (17.9)	525 (12.2)	1.6 (1.1–2.3)	0.02118	379 (22.4)	0.8 (0.5–1.1)	0.15263	47,086 (50.)	4.2 (2.9–6.0)	<0.001
HIV	3 (1.6)	158 (3.7)	0.4 (0.1–1.3)	0.12699	75 (4.4)	0.3 (0.1–1.1)	0.06099	8937 (0.9)	1.7 (0.5–5.3)	0.36796
Hodgkin's Disease	2 (1.1)	2 (0.0)	22.8 (3.2–162.7)	<0.001	2 (0.1)	9.0 (1.3–64.1)	0.00805	273 (0.0)	36.8 (9.1–148.9)	<0.001
Hyperlipidemia	48 (25.3)	961 (22.4)	1.2 (0.8–1.6)	0.35813	632 (37.4)	0.6 (0.4–0.8)	<0.001	72,033 (7.6)	4.1 (3.0–5.7)	<0.001
Hypertension	81 (42.6)	1333 (31.1)	1.6 (1.2–2.2)	<0.001	884 (52.3)	0.7 (0.5–0.9)	0.01141	127,879 (13.5)	4.7 (3.6–6.3)	<0.001
IBS	2 (1.1)	28 (0.7)	1.6 (0.4–6.8)	0.50894	18 (1.1)	1.0 (0.2–4.3)	0.98734	1363 (0.1)	7.4 (1.8–29.7)	<0.001
Ischemic Heart Disease	20 (10.5)	243 (5.7)	2.0 (1.2–3.2)	0.00533	183 (10.8)	1.0 (0.6–1.6)	0.89678	21,833 (2.3)	5.0 (3.1–7.9)	<0.001
Ischemic Stroke	7 (0.2)	0	0.57723	6 (0.4)	0	0.41072	847 (0.1)	0	0.6796	
Lung Cancer	1 (0.5)	8 (0.2)	2.8 (0.4–22.7)	0.30631	14 (0.8)	0.6 (0.1–4.8)	0.65722	1321 (0.1)	3.8 (0.5–27.0)	0.15429
Lymphomatoid Papulosis	1 (0.0)	0	0.83324					7 (0.0)	0	0.97006
Major Depressive Disorder	18 (9.5)	615 (14.3)	0.6 (0.4–1.0)	0.05928	265 (15.7)	0.6 (0.3–0.9)	0.0233	29,514 (3.1)	3.2 (2.0–5.3)	<0.001
Malignant Melanoma		3 (0.1)	0	0.71529				177 (0.0)	0	0.8503
Osteoarthritis	28 (14.7)	643 (15.0)	1.0 (0.7–1.5)	0.92114	433 (25.6)	0.5 (0.3–0.8)	<0.001	44,608 (4.7)	3.5 (2.3–5.2)	<0.001
Osteoporosis	2 (1.1)	83 (1.9)	0.5 (0.1–2.2)	0.38258	75 (4.4)	0.2 (0.1–0.9)	0.0256	5538 (0.6)	1.8 (0.4–7.3)	0.40015
Psoriasis	9 (4.7)	93 (2.2)	2.2 (1.1–4.5)	0.02029				1681 (0.2)	27.9 (14.2–54.5)	<0.001
Rheumatoid Arthritis	3 (1.6)	54 (1.3)	1.3 (0.4–4.1)	0.70085	60 (3.6)	0.4 (0.1–1.4)	0.15226	13,171 (1.4)	1.1 (0.4–3.5)	0.82869
Schizophrenia		53 (1.2)	0	0.12313	24 (1.4)	0	0.09829	5083 (0.5)	0	0.31056
Venous Thrombosis	10 (5.3)	114 (2.7)	2.0 (1.0–3.9)	0.03233	74 (4.4)	1.2 (0.6–2.4)	0.57583	9077 (1.)	5.7 (3.0–10.8)	<0.001
Vitamin D Deficiency	30 (15.8)	882 (20.6)	0.7 (0.5–1.1)	0.10909	433 (25.6)	0.5 (0.4–0.8)	0.00286	38,158 (4.0)	4.5 (3.0–6.6)	<0.001

Table A3. Absolute number, percentage, odds ratios and p values of White/Caucasian patients age 18 years and older with mycosis fungoides (MF) and various comorbid conditions, as compared with race-matched controls age 18 years and older with AD, with psoriasis, or within the general population who were seen at the JHHS between January 1, 2013 and January 1, 2019. Data presented for 329 patients with mycosis fungoides (MF), 4545 patients with AD, 11,700 patients with psoriasis, and 2,671,135 patients in the general population (excluding those with MF). AD, Atopic dermatitis; COPD, chronic obstructive pulmonary disease; OR, odds ratio; PN, prurigo nodularis; IBS, inflammatory bowel disease.

Comorbidity	MF, n (%)	AD, n (%)	OR (95% CI)	p Value	Psoriasis, n (%)	OR (95% CI)2	p Value	Gen Pop, n (%)	OR (95% CI)	p Value
Allergic Contact Dermatitis	4 (1.2)	249 (5.5)	0.2 (0.1–0.6)	<0.001	100 (0.9)	1.4 (0.5–3.9)	0.48534	3294 (0.1)	10.0 (3.7–26.7)	<0.001
Alzheimer Disease	3 (0.9)	15 (0.3)	2.8 (0.8–9.6)	0.09295	88 (0.8)	1.2 (0.4–3.9)	0.7416	6306 (0.2)	3.9 (1.2–12.1)	0.01157
Asthma	19 (5.8)	764 (16.8)	0.3 (0.2–0.5)	<0.001	1138 (9.7)	0.6 (0.4–0.9)	0.01651	58,241 (2.2)	2.7 (1.7–4.4)	<0.001
Atopic Dermatitis	11 (3.3)				224 (1.9)	1.8 (1.0–3.3)	0.06476	4534 (0.2)	20.3 (11.1–37.1)	<0.001

Table A3. Cont.

Comorbidity	MF, n (%)	AD, n (%)	OR (95% CI)	p Value	Psoriasis, n (%)	OR (95% CI)2	p Value	Gen Pop, n (%)	OR (95% CI)	p Value
Atrial Fibrillation	18 (5.5)	187 (4.1)	1.3 (0.8–2.2)	0.23646	808 (6.9)	0.8 (0.5–1.3)	0.31012	53,118 (2.0)	2.9 (1.8–4.6)	<0.001
Autistic Disorder		29 (0.6)	0	0.14617	10 (0.1)	0	0.59577	1451 (0.1)	0	0.67239
Breast Cancer		18 (0.4)	0	0.25279	62 (0.5)	0	0.18557	4966 (0.2)	0	0.43374
Chronic Hepatitis C	1 (0.3)	29 (0.6)	0.5 (0.1–3.5)	0.45432	137 (1.2)	0.3 (0.0–1.8)	0.14529	6140 (0.2)	1.3 (0.2–9.4)	0.7789
Chronic Kidney Disease	20 (6.1)	187 (4.1)	1.5 (0.9–2.4)	0.08793	707 (6.0)	1.0 (0.6–1.6)	0.97826	31,639 (1.2)	5.4 (3.4–8.5)	<0.001
Colon Cancer		4 (0.1)	0	0.59036	23 (0.2)	0	0.42083	1842 (0.1)	0	0.63373
Congestive Heart Failure	18 (5.5)	132 (2.9)	1.9 (1.2–3.2)	0.00924	518 (4.4)	1.2 (0.8–2.0)	0.3655	26,637 (1.0)	5.7 (3.6–9.2)	<0.001
COPD	21 (6.4)	209 (4.6)	1.4 (0.9–2.2)	0.14046	797 (6.8)	0.9 (0.6–1.5)	0.7605	35,482 (1.3)	5.1 (3.3–7.9)	<0.001
Diabetes Mellitus Type 2	24 (7.3)	346 (7.6)	1.0 (0.6–1.5)	0.83347	1562 (13.4)	0.5 (0.3–0.8)	0.00137	70,060 (2.6)	2.9 (1.9–4.4)	<0.001
HIV		18 (0.4)	0	0.25279	63 (0.5)	0	0.18204	3463 (0.1)	0	0.51342
Hodgkin's Disease	4 (1.2)	5 (0.1)	11.2 (3.0–41.8)	<0.001	16 (0.1)	9.0 (3.0–27.0)	<0.001	1103 (0.0)	29.8 (11.1–80.0)	<0.001
Hyperlipidemia	99 (30.1)	1408 (31.0)	1.0 (0.8–1.2)	0.73649	4631 (39.6)	0.7 (0.5–0.8)	<0.001	221,792 (8.3)	4.8 (3.8–6.0)	<0.001
Hypertension	102 (31.0)	1337 (29.4)	1.1 (0.8–1.4)	0.5425	4733 (40.5)	0.7 (0.5–0.8)	<0.001	251,808 (9.4)	4.3 (3.4–5.5)	<0.001
IBS	2 (0.6)	50 (1.1)	0.5 (0.1–2.3)	0.40138	198 (1.7)	0.4 (0.1–1.4)	0.12925	6582 (0.2)	2.5 (0.6–9.9)	0.18606
Ischemic Heart Disease	29 (8.8)	224 (4.9)	1.9 (1.2–2.8)	0.00215	995 (8.5)	1.0 (0.7–1.5)	0.84233	50,371 (1.9)	5.0 (3.4–7.4)	<0.001
Ischemic Stroke	-	14 (0.3)	0	0.31339	28 (0.2)	0	0.37435	1564 (0.1)	0	0.66064
Lung Cancer	2 (0.6)	16 (0.4)	1.7 (0.4–7.6)	0.46001	65 (0.6)	1.1 (0.3–4.5)	0.89987	5063 (0.2)	3.2 (0.8–12.9)	0.08111
Lymphomatoid Papulosis	10 (3.0)	3 (0.1)	47.5 (13.0–173.3)	<0.001				39 (0.0)	2147.0 (1062.6–4338.1)	<0.001
Major Depressive Disorder	25 (7.6)	617 (13.6)	0.5 (0.3–0.8)	0.00197	1720 (14.7)	0.5 (0.3–0.7)	<0.001	80,063 (3.0)	2.7 (1.8–4.0)	<0.001
Malignant Melanoma	9 (2.7)	65 (1.4)	1.9 (1.0–3.9)	0.0615	157 (1.3)	2.1 (1.0–4.1)	0.03259	7314 (0.3)	10.2 (3.7–26.7)	<0.001
Osteoarthritis	48 (14.6)	869 (19.1)	0.7 (0.5–1.0)	0.04233	3281 (28.0)	0.4 (0.3–0.6)	<0.001	125,515 (4.7)	3.5 (2.6–4.7)	<0.001
Osteoporosis	10 (3.0)	261 (5.7)	0.5 (0.3–1.0)	0.03882	729 (6.2)	0.5 (0.3–0.9)	0.01744	33,605 (1.3)	2.5 (1.3–4.6)	0.00375
Psoriasis	12 (3.6)	224 (4.9)	0.7 (0.4–1.3)	0.29586				11,689 (0.4)	8.6 (4.8–15.3)	<0.001
Rheumatoid Arthritis	5 (1.5)	58 (1.3)	1.2 (0.5–3.0)	0.70559	390 (3.3)	0.4 (0.2–1.1)	0.06869	35,498 (1.3)	1.1 (0.5–2.8)	0.76249
Schizophrenia	2 (0.6)	16 (0.4)	1.7 (0.4–7.6)	0.46001	43 (0.4)	1.7 (0.4–6.9)	0.4812	2777 (0.1)	5.9 (1.5–23.6)	0.00458
Venous Thrombosis	12 (3.6)	130 (2.9)	1.3 (0.7–2.3)	0.41235	403 (3.4)	1.1 (0.6–1.9)	0.84231	22,078 (0.8)	4.5 (2.6–8.1)	<0.001
Vitamin D Deficiency	29 (8.8)	838 (18.4)	0.4 (0.3–0.6)	<0.001	2259 (19.3)	0.4 (0.3–0.6)	<0.001	75,560 (2.8)	3.3 (2.3–4.9)	<0.001

References

1. Song, S.X.; Willemze, R.; Swerdlow, S.H.; Kinney, M.C.; Said, J.W. Mycosis fungoides: Report of the 2011 Society for Hematopathology/European Association for Haematopathology workshop. *Am. J. Clin. Pathol.* **2013**, *139*, 466–490. [CrossRef] [PubMed]
2. Jawed, S.I.; Myskowski, P.L.; Horwitz, S.; Moskowitz, A.; Querfeld, C. Primary cutaneous T-cell lymphoma (mycosis fungoides and Sezary syndrome): Part I. Diagnosis: Clinical and histopathologic features and new molecular and biologic markers. *J. Am. Acad. Dermatol.* **2014**, *70*, e1–e16. [CrossRef] [PubMed]
3. Criscione, V.D.; Weinstock, M.A. Incidence of cutaneous T-cell lymphoma in the United States, 1973–2002. *Arch. Dermatol.* **2007**, *143*, 854–859. [CrossRef] [PubMed]
4. Korgavkar, K.; Xiong, M.; Weinstock, M. Changing incidence trends of cutaneous T-cell lymphoma. *JAMA Dermatol.* **2013**, *149*, 1295–1299. [CrossRef] [PubMed]
5. Nikolaou, V.; Marinos, L.; Moustou, E.; Papadavid, E.; Economidi, A.; Christofidou, E.; Gerochristou, M.; Tasidou, A.; Economaki, E.; Stratigos, A.; et al. Psoriasis in patients with mycosis fungoides: A clinicopathological study of 25 patients. *J. Eur. Acad. Dermatol. Venereol.* **2017**, *31*, 1848–1852. [CrossRef]
6. El Tawdy, A.M.; Amin, I.M.; Abdel Hay, R.M.; Hassan, A.S.; Gad, Z.S.; Rashed, L.A. Toll-like receptor (TLR)7 expression in mycosis fungoides and psoriasis: A case-control study. *Clin. Exp. Dermatol.* **2017**, *42*, 172–177. [CrossRef]
7. Cengiz, F.P.; Emiroglu, N. Evaluation of cardiovascular disease risk factors in patients with mycosis fungoides. *An. Bras. Dermatol.* **2015**, *90*, 36–40. [CrossRef]
8. Kim, Y.H.; Liu, H.L.; Mraz-Gernhard, S.; Varghese, A.; Hoppe, R.T. Long-term outcome of 525 patients with mycosis fungoides and Sezary syndrome: Clinical prognostic factors and risk for disease progression. *Arch. Dermatol.* **2003**, *139*, 857–866. [CrossRef]
9. Lindahl, L.M.; Fenger-Gron, M.; Iversen, L. Subsequent cancers, mortality, and causes of death in patients with mycosis fungoides and parapsoriasis: A Danish nationwide, population-based cohort study. *J. Am. Acad. Dermatol.* **2014**, *71*, 529–535. [CrossRef]
10. Boozalis, E.; Tang, O.; Patel, S.; Semenov, Y.R.; Pereira, M.P.; Stander, S.; Kang, S.; Kwatra, S.G. Ethnic differences and comorbidities of 909 prurigo nodularis patients. *J. Am. Acad. Dermatol.* **2018**, *79*, 714–719. [CrossRef]
11. Larson, V.A.; Tang, O.; Stander, S.; Kang, S.; Kwatra, S.G. Association between itch and cancer in 16,925 patients with pruritus: Experience at a tertiary care center. *J. Am. Acad. Dermatol.* **2019**, *80*, 931–937. [CrossRef] [PubMed]
12. Govind, K.; Whang, K.; Khanna, R.; Scott, A.W.; Kwatra, S.G. Atopic dermatitis is associated with increased prevalence of multiple ocular comorbidities. *J. Allergy Clin. Immunol. Pract.* **2019**, *7*, 298–299. [CrossRef] [PubMed]
13. Chronic Conditions. US Centers for Medicare and Medicaid Services. Available online: https://www.cms.gov/Research-Statistics-Data-and-Systems/Statistics-Trends-and-Reports/Chronic-Conditions/CC_Main.html (accessed on 27 December 2017).
14. Morales Suarez-Varela, M.M.; Llopis Gonzalez, A.; Marquina Vila, A.; Bell, J. Mycosis fungoides: Review of epidemiological observations. *Dermatology* **2000**, *201*, 21–28. [CrossRef] [PubMed]
15. Lim, H.L.J.; Tan, E.S.T.; Tee, S.I.; Ho, Z.Y.; Boey, J.J.J.; Tan, W.P.; Tang, M.B.Y.; Shen, L.; Chan, Y.H.; Tan, S.H. Epidemiology and prognostic factors for mycosis fungoides and Sezary syndrome in a multi-ethnic Asian cohort: A 12-year review. *J. Eur. Acad. Dermatol. Venereol.* **2019**, *33*, 1513–1521. [CrossRef]
16. Amorim, G.M.; Niemeyer-Corbellini, J.P.; Quintella, D.C.; Cuzzi, T.; Ramos-E-Silva, M. Clinical and epidemiological profile of patients with early stage mycosis fungoides. *An. Bras. Dermatol.* **2018**, *93*, 546–552. [CrossRef]
17. Su, C.; Nguyen, K.A.; Bai, H.X.; Cao, Y.; Tao, Y.; Xiao, R.; Karakousis, G.; Zhang, P.J.; Zhang, G. Racial disparity in mycosis fungoides: An analysis of 4495 cases from the US National Cancer Database. *J. Am. Acad. Dermatol.* **2017**, *77*, 497–502. [CrossRef]
18. Larocca, C.; Kupper, T. Mycosis fungoides and Sezary syndrome: An update. *Hematol. Oncol. Clin. N. Am.* **2019**, *33*, 103–120. [CrossRef]
19. Imam, M.H.; Shenoy, P.J.; Flowers, C.R.; Phillips, A.; Lechowicz, M.J. Incidence and survival patterns of cutaneous T-cell lymphomas in the United States. *Leuk. Lymphoma* **2013**, *54*, 752–759. [CrossRef]

20. Huang, A.H.; Kwatra, S.G.; Khanna, R.; Semenov, Y.R.; Okoye, G.A.; Sweren, R.J. Racial disparities in the clinical presentation and prognosis of patients with mycosis fungoides. *J. Natl. Med. Assoc.* **2019**, *111*, 633–639. [CrossRef]
21. Wieser, I.; Oh, C.W.; Talpur, R.; Duvic, M. Lymphomatoid papulosis: Treatment response and associated lymphomas in a study of 180 patients. *J. Am. Acad. Dermatol.* **2016**, *74*, 59–67. [CrossRef]
22. Huang, K.P.; Weinstock, M.A.; Clarke, C.A.; McMillan, A.; Hoppe, R.T.; Kim, Y.H. Second lymphomas and other malignant neoplasms in patients with mycosis fungoides and Sezary syndrome: Evidence from population-based and clinical cohorts. *Arch. Dermatol.* **2007**, *143*, 45–50. [CrossRef] [PubMed]
23. Hallermann, C.; Kaune, K.M.; Tiemann, M.; Kunze, E.; Griesinger, F.; Mitteldorf, C.; Bertsch, H.P.; Neumann, C. High frequency of primary cutaneous lymphomas associated with lymphoproliferative disorders of different lineage. *Ann. Hematol.* **2007**, *86*, 509–515. [CrossRef] [PubMed]
24. Amber, K.T.; Bloom, R.; Nouri, K. Second primary malignancies in CTCL patients from 1992 to 2011: A SEER-based, population-based study evaluating time from CTCL diagnosis, age, sex, stage, and CD30+ subtype. *Am. J. Clin. Dermatol.* **2016**, *17*, 71–77. [CrossRef] [PubMed]
25. AbuHilal, M.; Walsh, S.; Shear, N. associated hematolymphoid malignancies in patients with lymphomatoid papulosis: A Canadian retrospective study. *J. Cutan. Med. Surg.* **2017**, *21*, 507–512. [CrossRef]
26. Hodak, E.; Lessin, S.; Friedland, R.; Freud, T.; David, M.; Pavlovsky, L.; Shapiro, J.; Cohen, A.D. New insights into associated co-morbidities in patients with cutaneous T-cell lymphoma (mycosis fungoides). *Acta Derm. Venereol.* **2013**, *93*, 451–455. [CrossRef]
27. Smoller, B.R.; Marcus, R. Risk of secondary cutaneous malignancies in patients with long-standing mycosis fungoides. *J. Am. Acad. Dermatol.* **1994**, *30*, 201–204. [CrossRef]
28. Lutsyk, M.; Ben-Yosef, R.; Bergman, R.; Kuten, A.; Bar-Sela, G. Total Skin Electron Irradiation and Sequential Malignancies in Mycosis Fungoides Patients: Longitudinal Study. *Clin. Oncol.* **2018**, *30*, 618–624. [CrossRef]
29. Legendre, L.; Barnetche, T.; Mazereeuw-Hautier, J.; Meyer, N.; Murrell, D.; Paul, C. Risk of lymphoma in patients with atopic dermatitis and the role of topical treatment: A systematic review and meta-analysis. *J. Am. Acad. Dermatol.* **2015**, *72*, 992–1002. [CrossRef]
30. Kechichian, E.; Ezzedine, K. Vitamin D and the Skin: An update for dermatologists. *Am. J. Clin. Dermatol.* **2018**, *19*, 223–235. [CrossRef]
31. Talpur, R.; Cox, K.M.; Hu, M.; Geddes, E.R.; Parker, M.K.; Yang, B.Y.; Armstrong, P.A.; Liu, P.; Duvic, M. Vitamin D deficiency in mycosis fungoides and Sezary syndrome patietns is smiilar to other cancer patients. *Clin. Lymphoma Myeloma Leuk.* **2014**, *14*, 518–524. [CrossRef]
32. Joseph, P.; Leong, D.; McKee, M.; Anand, S.S.; Schwalm, J.D.; Teo, K.; Mente, A.; Yusuf, S. Reducing the global burden of cardiovascular disease, Part 1: The epidemiology AND risk factors. *Circ. Res.* **2017**, *121*, 677–694. [CrossRef] [PubMed]

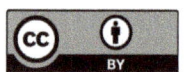

© 2019 by the authors. Licensee MDPI, Basel, Switzerland. This article is an open access article distributed under the terms and conditions of the Creative Commons Attribution (CC BY) license (http://creativecommons.org/licenses/by/4.0/).

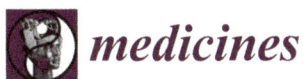

Article

Association between Itch and Cancer in 3836 Pediatric Pruritus Patients at a Tertiary Care Center

Micah Belzberg [1], Valerie A. Larson [1], Raveena Khanna [1], Kyle A. Williams [1], Yevgeniy Semenov [2], Sonja Ständer [3], Anna L. Grossberg [1] and Shawn G. Kwatra [1,4,*

[1] Department of Dermatology, Johns Hopkins University School of Medicine, Baltimore, MD 21231, USA; mbelzbe@jhu.edu (M.B.); vgordon4@jhmi.edu (V.A.L.); rkhanna8@jhmi.edu (R.K.); kwill184@health.fau.edu (K.A.W.); agrossb2@jhmi.edu (A.L.G.)
[2] Dermatology, Washington University School of Medicine, St. Louis, MO 63110, USA; yevgeniy.semenov1@gmail.com
[3] Center for Chronic Pruritus, Department of Dermatology, University Hospital Münster, 48149 Münster, Germany; Sonja.Staender@ukmuenster.de
[4] Bloomberg School of Public Health, Johns Hopkins Bloomberg School of Public Health, Baltimore, MD 21205, USA
* Correspondence: skwatra1@jhmi.edu; Tel.: +1-410-955-8662

Received: 21 August 2019; Accepted: 26 September 2019; Published: 5 October 2019

Abstract: Background: Pruritus is a well-recognized paraneoplastic phenomenon. Previous studies have examined the association of itch with a variety of malignancies in adults. However, no large study has examined this association in a pediatric population. **Methods**: A retrospective study was conducted of patients age 18 or less seen at Johns Hopkins Health System between 2012 and 2019. **Results**: A pediatric hospital population of 1,042,976 patients was reviewed. Pruritus was observed in 3836 pediatric patients of whom 130 also had cancer. Pediatric patients with pruritus were significantly more likely to have concomitant malignancy compared to pediatric patients without pruritus (OR 12.84; 95% CI 10.73–15.35, $p < 0.001$). Malignancies most strongly associated with pruritus included neoplasms of the blood (OR 14.38; 95% CI 11.30–18.29, $p < 0.001$), bone (OR 29.02, 95% CI 18.28–46.06, $p < 0.001$) and skin (OR 22.76, 95% CI 9.14–56.72, $p < 0.001$. **Conclusions**: Pruritus is significantly associated with malignancy in the pediatric hospital population. Clinicians should also be aware of the high burden of itch in pediatric malignancies and the variation in pruritus across malignancies.

Keywords: itch; pruritus; pediatric; children; malignancy; cancer; neoplasm; epidemiology

1. Introduction

Pruritus is a well-recognized phenomenon in cancer [1]. Previous studies have examined the association of itch or pruritic dermatosis with a variety of malignancies in the adult population [2–5]. However, the pediatric population experiences significantly different ratios of malignancy types, such as higher fractions of hematologic and nervous system related cancers [6,7]. We therefore expect the association of pruritus and malignancy to be different in the pediatric population.

Sporadic case reports have presented pediatric patients with pruritus who upon investigation were subsequently diagnosed with malignancies [8–12]. However, to our knowledge, no study has examined the association of itch and cancer or the types of underlying cancers associated with itch in a pediatric population. The objective of this study was therefore to examine the association of pruritus and malignancy in pediatric patients at a USA tertiary care center.

2. Materials and Methods

A retrospective study was conducted of pediatric patients seen at Johns Hopkins Health System (JHHS), a U.S. tertiary care center which draws a diverse range of local, regional, national, and international patients. The study population consisted of all patients age 18 or less seen at JHHS between 1 January 2012 and 1 January 2019. Anonymized aggregate-level data was collected using the Slicer Dicer function within Johns Hopkins EPIC electronic medical records [3–5,13,14]. IRB approval was therefore waived. SNOMED-CT concept terms were used to specify all data [3–5,13,14]. All results combined male and female patients.

2.1. Pediatric Pruritus Population

Using an EPIC Slicer Dicer, 3809 pediatric patients with a visit diagnosis, billing diagnosis, or active problem list entry of "itching" were identified [3]. The comparison group was 1,039,167 pediatric patients without pruritus seen at JHHS over the same period. Each case of pruritus was also subdivided into patients with or without a skin eruption ("eruption of skin").

2.2. Pediatric Cancer Population

An EPIC Slicer Dicer was used to identify all pediatric patients with a diagnosed primary malignant neoplasm (PMN). Malignancies were grouped by organ or organ system. Hematologic malignancies were further delineated using disease specific diagnoses. Separately, patients were identified in whom pruritus was diagnosed within the six months preceding their diagnosis of malignancy.

2.3. Statistical Analyses

Analyses compared instances of malignancy in pediatric patients with or without pruritus. Additional analyses examined instances of pruritus in each malignancy. Sub analyses were performed examining racial variation, age distribution, and the presence of concurrent kidney disease, liver disease, hyperbilirubinemia, endocrine disorders and antineoplastic medication treatment. Microsoft Excel (Redmond, WA, USA) was used to calculate odds ratios and 95% confidence intervals. Chi-squared statistics with one degree of freedom were used to calculate odds ratio p-values. Z-tests were used to calculate p-values for comparisons of odds ratios. To account for multiple comparisons, a Bonferroni correction was applied to the alpha level for each analysis (alpha = 0.05/[number of independent comparisons]).

3. Results

Between 2012 and 2019, a total of 1,042,976 pediatric patients were seen at JHHS. Demographic data are presented in Table 1. The distribution of primary malignancies identified in the pediatric hospital population is summarized in Figure 1.

Table 1. Patient demographics.

Characteristic	All (n = 1,042,976) n (%)	Itching (n = 3836) n (%)	All PMNs (n = 2980) n (%)	PMNs + Itching (n = 130) n (%)
Sex				
Male	542,125 (52)	1542 (40)	1571 (53)	65 (50)
Female	504,788 (48)	2302 (60)	1409 (47)	65 (50)
Race				
White/Caucasian	515,696 (49)	1348 (35)	1539 (52)	73 (56)
Black/African American	263,166 (25)	1771 (46)	567 (19)	27 (20)
Asian	51,847 (5)	202(5)	145 (5)	10 (8)
Age Range				
0–6	292,033 (28)	1151(30)	805 (27)	42 (32)
6–12	365,042 (35)	1458 (38)	1013(34)	43 (33)
12–18	385,901 (37)	1228 (32)	1162 (39)	45 (35)

Sex, race, and age distribution of the study population and study subgroups. Primary malignant neoplasm (PMN).

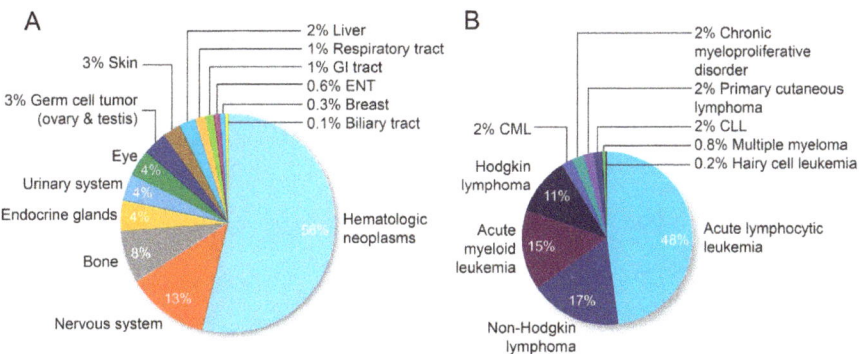

Figure 1. Distribution of malignancies in the pediatric population at JHHS. (**A**) Frequency of each malignancy subtype among patients age 18 or less. (**B**) Breakdown of blood malignancies as a percentage of total hematologic cancers. Chronic myeloid leukemia (CML) and Chronic lymphoid leukemia (CLL).

3.1. Pruritus Is Strongly Associated with Malignancy in the Pediatric Population

Between 2019 and 2012, 3809 pediatric patients with itching were treated at JHHS of whom 130 were diagnosed with a concomitant malignancy. Pediatric patients with itching were significantly more likely than pediatric patients without a diagnosis of itching to have malignancy (OR 12.84; 95% CI 10.73–15.35, $p < 0.001$) (Figure 2). PMNs strongly associated with pruritus included neoplasms of bone (OR 29.02; 95% CI 18.28–46.46, $p < 0.001$), skin (OR 22.76, 95% CI 9.14–13.63, $p < 0.001$), liver (OR 21.55; 95% CI 6.65–14.9, $p < 0.001$), and blood (OR 14.38; 95% CI 11.30–18.29, $p < 0.001$). Among hematologic dyscrasias, diagnoses most strongly associated with pruritus included acute myeloid leukemia (OR 23.14; 95% CI 14.64–36.56, $p < 0.001$), Hodgkin lymphoma (OR 12.35, 95% CI 6.08–25.11 $p < 0.001$), non–Hodgkin lymphoma (OR 10.48; 95% CI 5.74–19.16, $p < 0.001$), and acute lymphocytic leukemia (OR 10.47; 95% CI 7.26–15.10, $p < 0.001$). The weakest association was observed for neoplasms of the nervous system (OR 1.26; 95% CI 2.13 5.70, $p = 0.009$), and eye (OR 2.87; 95% CI 0.40–20.61, $p = 0.27$). No pruritus was observed in PMNs of the germ cells or biliary tract.

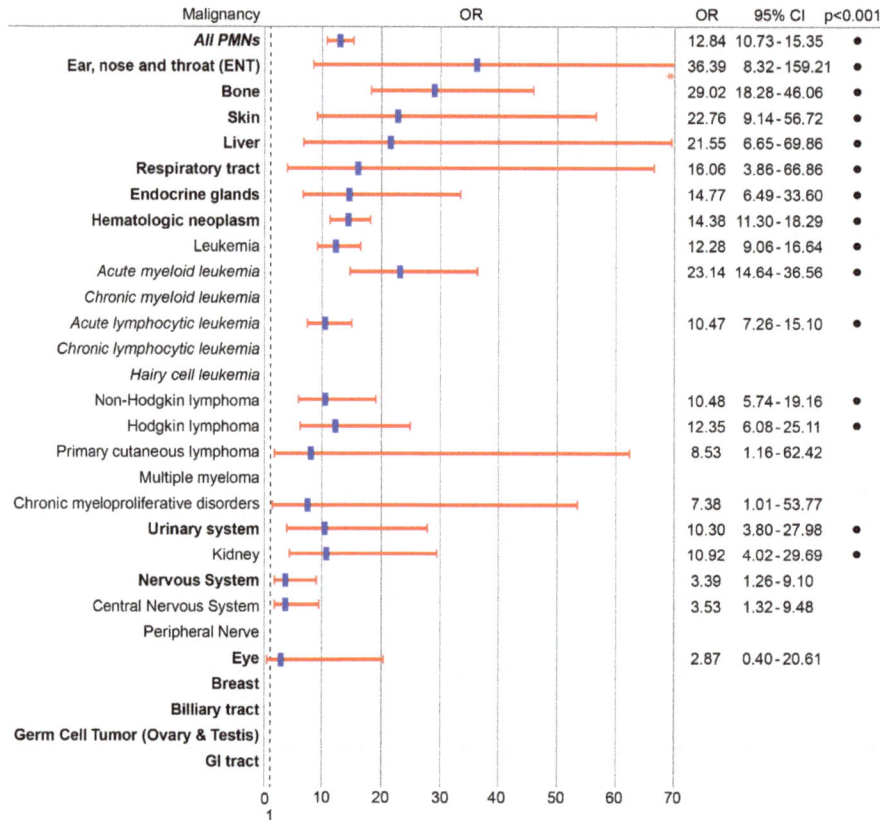

Figure 2. Itching is strongly associated with pediatric malignancies. Odds ratio (OR) with 95% confidence interval (95% CI) of malignancy in patients with compared to without itching in the general pediatric hospital population. Blank rows denote malignancies for which there were no concurrent diagnoses of pruritus. * 95% CI upper limit for ENT (159.2) has been truncated. • = $p < 0.001$, chi-squared test. Primary malignant neoplasm (PMN).

3.2. Racial Variation

Racial variation was observed in the association of pruritus and malignancy; however, upon further analyses, this variation appeared driven by racial differences in malignancy rates. Compared to Whites/Caucasians, Blacks/African Americans had significantly lower prevalence of certain neoplasms including bone, endocrine, and blood cancers. Rates of pruritus within individual malignancies were not significantly different between races.

3.3. The Prevalence of Skin Eruptions Varies with Underlying Malignancy

Of the 3836 pediatric patients diagnosed with itching, 767 (20%) were also diagnosed with an eruption of skin. Among the 130 pediatric patients diagnosed with pruritus and malignancy, a skin eruption was observed in 34 instances (26%). The highest prevalence of skin eruption amongst pediatric patients with pruritus and malignancy were observed in PMNs of ear, nose, and throat (ENT) (100%), endocrine glands (50%), blood (35%), and bone (30%) (Figure 3). Amongst blood neoplasms, the highest prevalence was observed in Hodgkin lymphoma (63%) and leukemia (40%). No incidences of skin eruption concurrent to pruritus were observed with PMNs of the liver, nervous system, or skin.

Odds ratio comparison revealed the prevalence of itching with skin eruption was significantly higher among hematologic cancers when compared to non-hematologic malignancies (OR 3.02, 95% CI 1.28–7.14, $p < 0.01$).

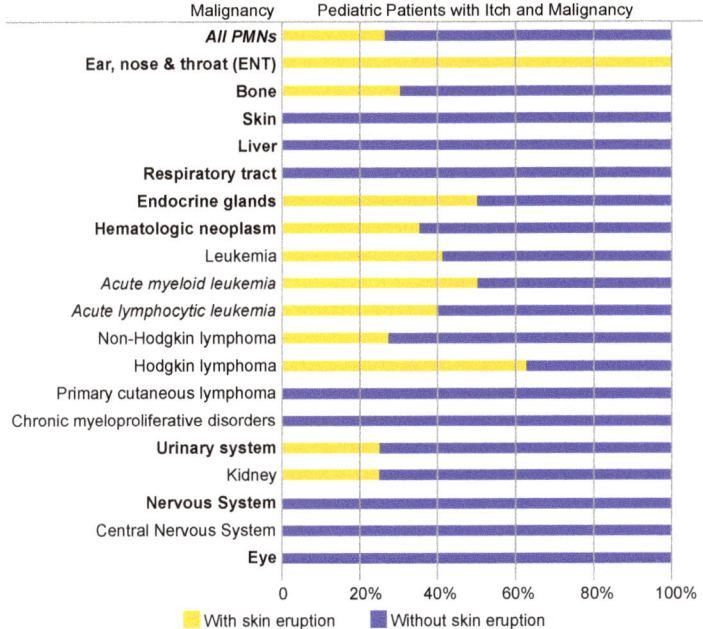

Figure 3. Prevalence of skin eruption in pediatric patients with itch and malignancy is variable. Lighter bars denote the percentage of patients with pruritus and a primary malignant neoplasm (PMN) who had a concurrent skin eruption. Darker bars denote percentage of patients with pruritus and a PMN without concurrent skin eruption.

3.4. Pruritus Preceding Malignancy Is Associated with Hematologic Malignancy

Out of the total study population, 17 cases were identified in which a diagnosis of pruritus was made in the six months preceding a diagnosis of malignancy. Itch most often preadded PMNs of blood (7/17, 41%) and the gastrointestinal tract (2/17, 12%). The most frequently-diagnosed hematologic neoplasms were leukemia (3/17, 18%) and non-Hodgkin lymphoma (3/17, 18%).

3.5. Pruritus Among Pediatric Cancer Patients Is Associated with Comorbid Kidney Disease, Liver Disease, and Antineoplastic Use

Analyses of pediatric patients with malignancy and itch found a statistically significant ($p < 0.01$) increased incidence of concurrent kidney disease, liver disease, and antineoplastic medication use when compared to pediatric patients with malignancy but without itch (Figure 4). The subset of pediatric patients with PMNs and itching accompanied by skin eruption showed a statistically significant ($p < 0.01$) increased prevalence of hyperbilirubinemia, kidney disease, and antineoplastic use when compared with pediatric patients with cancer but without pruritus. The prevalence of these comorbidities in patients with pruritus within six months prior to their PMN diagnoses did not reach statistical significance.

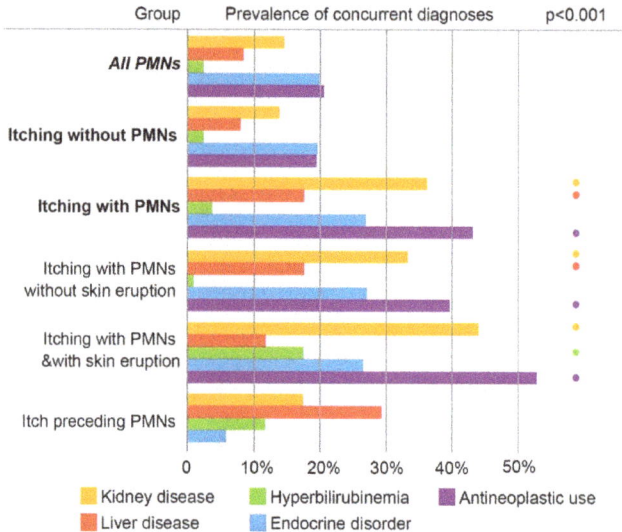

Figure 4. Pruritus among pediatric cancer patients is associated with comorbidities. Percentages of each group with concurrent diagnoses of kidney disease (gold), liver disease (red), hyperbilirubinemia (green), antineoplastic use (purple), and endocrine disorders (blue). • denotes statistically significant difference in comorbidity prevalence compared to pediatric patients with a primary malignant neoplasm (PMN) but without itch ($p < 0.01$).

4. Discussion

Pruritus is known to be associated with malignancies in adults, however limited data is available in the pediatric population [1,2]. While there have been sporadic pediatric cases of itch associated with diagnosed neoplasms, no large study has examined this association within a pediatric population [8–12]. Our findings demonstrate associations between pruritus and malignancy in a diverse pediatric population at a USA tertiary care center.

Compared to pediatric patients without itch, pediatric patients with itch were 13 times more likely to also be diagnosed with a malignancy (OR 12.84; 95% CI 10.73–15.35). By contrast, in a previous study examining the association of itch and malignancy in the adult population, patients 18 years or older with pruritus were approximately six times more likely to have concurrent malignancy as compared to adult patients without pruritus (OR 5.76; 95% CI 5.53–6.00) [3].

In the present study, the association of pruritus and malignancy was strongest for PMNs of bone, skin, liver, and blood, in particular, leukemia, non-Hodgkin and Hodgkin lymphoma. The association was weakest amongst PMNs of the eye and nervous system. These findings somewhat differ from those observed in adult patients with cancer. In the adult population, strong associations between itch and malignancy were observed in PMNs of liver, blood, and skin with weaker associations in PMNs of bone [3].

Previous publications have presented cases of pediatric patients with unexplained itch who upon investigation were subsequently diagnosed with neoplasms such as Hodgkin lymphoma, Non-Hodgkin lymphoma, T-cell lymphoma, and hepatocellular carcinoma [8–12]. In adults, pruritus has been observed to most frequently proceed a hematologic malignancy or occasionally gastric cancers [15,16]. This study identified 17 pediatric patients with pruritus preceding their diagnoses of malignancy. Most often these pediatric pruritic patients were later diagnosed with hematologic neoplasms (7/17, 41%). Two instances of pruritus preceding gastric malignancy were also observed. These findings suggest pediatric patients with itch and possible malignancy receive appropriate work up for hematologic neoplasms.

Subgroup analyses stratified by race revealed pronounced variation in the association of itch and malignancy. However, further analyses revealed rates of pruritus in categorical malignancies were not significantly different between races. The observed variation in association is therefore most likely due to racial differences in malignancy rates and not due to racial differences in pruritus.

The pathophysiology of pruritus in malignancy remains poorly understood [15,17]. Multiple etiologies have been described including systemic inflammation, local mass effect, antineoplastic medication use, and disruption of the hepatic or renal systems [15,18]. Hepatobiliary involvement may induce itch via accumulation of bile salts, bile acids, and bilirubin or perhaps through increased opiodergic tone [15,18,19]. Kidney invasion, ureteric obstruction, or renal failure meanwhile may induce uremic itch via the accumulation of pruritogenic metabolites or possibly a cytokine imbalance [15]. With respect to the pathogenesis of pruritus in hematologic malignancies, several mechanisms have been proposed. Previous studies have pointed to a possible role of opioid receptors owing to the observed efficacy of butorphanol in reducing pruritus in a patient with non-Hodgkin lymphoma [15,20]. Alternatively, variations in cytokine expression, known to be increased in atopic dermatitis, have also been observed in patients with both Hodgkin and non-Hodgkin lymphomas [15,21,22].

Compared to pediatric patients with malignancy but without itch, pediatric patients with PMNs and pruritus were observed to have significantly higher prevalence of kidney disease, liver disease, and antineoplastic medication use. Alternatively, patients with malignancy and itching with skin eruption showed significantly increased prevalence of hyperbilirubinemia, kidney disease, and antineoplastic use. These findings align with previously proposed mechanisms of pruritus in malignancy [15,17,18]. Additional analyses are needed to determine if these comorbidities developed as a direct result of a primary neoplastic process or secondary to antineoplastic use. Furthermore, additional studies are needed to examine the specific qualities of pruritis in malignancies and compare variation in itch intensity, location, and duration between different malignancy types.

Significant differences in pruritus rates were observed between malignancies of different systems as well as between individual malignancy types. The reason for this variation is likely multifactorial including differences in therapeutic management and effect on hepatic or renal processes [15,17,18]. With respect to hematologic malignancies, this observed variation may also be driven by differences in cytokine expression [21–24]. Additionally, very few incidences of certain cancers including hairy cell leukemia, multiple myeloma, and breast cancer were observed in our pediatric population which may limit these findings.

Data were collected through a retrospective design therefore the cause–effect relationship of these findings is limited. The tertiary care center population studied may limit the generalizability of these findings to different populations. Additional unknown confounders such as differences in socioeconomic level or other medical comorbidities could further limit these results.

5. Conclusions

In summary, our results indicate that pruritus is strongly associated with malignancy in the pediatric population. Malignancies strongly associated included PMNs of bone, skin, liver, endocrine glands, and blood. Additionally, several instances of itch preceding malignancy were identified. To improve patient management and diagnosis, clinicians should recognize the high burden of itch in pediatric malignancies and the variation in pruritus association across different malignancies.

Author Contributions: Study was conceptualized by M.B., V.A.L. and S.G.K. Study methodology was developed with contributions by all authors (M.B., V.A.L., R.K., K.A.W., Y.S., S.S., A.L.G. and S.G.K.). Data analyses was performed by M.B., V.A.L., R.K. and S.G.K. Original draft preparation, review and editing was performed by all authors (M.B., V.A.L., R.K., K.A.W., Y.S., S.S., A.L.G. and S.G.K.). Data visualization was performed by M.B., V.A.L. and S.G.K. Project supervision and administration was performed by Y.S., S.S., A.L.G. and S.G.K.

Funding: This research received no external funding.

Conflicts of Interest: S.G.K. is an advisory board member for Menlo and Trevi Therapeutics.

References

1. Rowe, B.; Yosipovitch, G. Malignancy-associated pruritus. *Eur. J. Pain* **2016**, *20*, 19–23. [CrossRef] [PubMed]
2. Kilic, A.; Gul, U.; Soylu, S. Skin findings in internal malignant diseases. *Int. J. Dermatol.* **2007**, *46*, 1055–1060. [CrossRef]
3. Larson, V.A.; Tang, O.; Stander, S.; Kang, S.; Kwatra, S.G. Association between itch and cancer in 16,925 patients with pruritus: Experience at a tertiary care center. *J. Am. Acad. Dermatol.* **2019**, *80*, 931–937. [CrossRef] [PubMed]
4. Larson, V.A.; Tang, O.; Stander, S.; Miller, L.S.; Kang, S.; Kwatra, S.G. Association between prurigo nodularis and malignancy in middle-aged adults. *J. Am. Acad. Dermatol.* **2019**. [CrossRef]
5. Huang, A.H.; Canner, J.K.; Khanna, R.; Kang, S.; Kwatra, S.G. Real-world prevalence of prurigo nodularis and burden of associated diseases. *J. Investig. Dermatol.* **2019**. [CrossRef]
6. Jemal, A.; Siegel, R.; Ward, E.; Hao, Y.; Xu, J.; Thun, M.J. Cancer statistics, 2019. *CA Cancer J. Clin.* **2019**, *69*, 7–34. [CrossRef]
7. Steliarova-Foucher, E.; Colombet, M.; Ries, L.A.; Moreno, F.; Dolya, A.; Bray, F.; Hesseling, P.; Shin, H.Y.; Stiller, S.A. International incidence of childhood cancer, 2001-10: A population-based registry study. *Lancet Oncol.* **2017**, *18*, 719–731. [CrossRef]
8. De la Bretèque Amy, M.; Bilan, P.; Galesowski, A.; Chevallier, B.; Drouot, D.; Sigal, M.L.; Mahé, E. Two cases of severe pruritus revealing Hodgkin's disease in children. *Annales de Dermatologie et de Venereologie* **2014**, *141*, 765–768. [CrossRef]
9. Vècsei, A.; Attarbaschi, A.; Krammer, U.; Mann, G.; Gadner, H. Pruritus in pediatric non-Hodgkin's lymphoma. *Leuk. Lymphoma* **2002**, *43*, 1885–1887. [CrossRef] [PubMed]
10. Hon, K.L.E.; Lam, M.C.A.; Leung, T.F.; Chik, K.W.; Leung, A.K. A malignant itch. *J. Natl. Med. Assoc.* **2006**, *98*, 1992–1994.
11. Vilarinho, S.; Erson-Omay, E.Z.; Harmanci, A.S.; Morotti, R.; Carrion-Grant, G.; Baranoski, J.; Knisely, A.S.; Ekong, U.; Emre, S.; Yasuno, K.; et al. Paediatric hepatocellular carcinoma due to somatic CTNNB1 and NFE2L2 mutations in the setting of inherited bi-allelic ABCB11 mutations. *J. Hepatol.* **2014**, *61*, 1178–1183. [CrossRef] [PubMed]
12. Tonnhofer, U.; Balassy, C.; Reck, C.A.; Koller, A.; Horcher, E. Neuroendocrine tumor of the common hepatic duct, mimicking a choledochal cyst in a 6-year-old child. *J. Pediatric. Surg.* **2009**, *44*, 23–25. [CrossRef] [PubMed]
13. Govind, K.; Whang, K.; Khanna, R.; Scott, A.W.; Kwatra, S.G. Atopic dermatitis is associated with increased prevalence of multiple ocular comorbidities. *J. Allergy Clin. Immunol. Pract.* **2019**, *7*, 298–299. [CrossRef] [PubMed]
14. Boozalis, E.; Tang, O.; Patel, S.; Semenov, Y.R.; Pereira, M.P.; Stander, S.; Kang, S.; Kwatra, S.G. Ethnic differences and comorbidities of 909 prurigo nodularis patients. *J. Am. Acad. Dermatol.* **2018**, *79*, 714–719. [CrossRef]
15. Yosipovitch, G. Chronic pruritus: A paraneoplastic sign. *Dermatol. Ther.* **2010**, *23*, 590–596. [CrossRef]
16. Zirwas, M.J.; Seraly, M.P. Pruritus of unknown origin: A retrospective study. *J. Am. Acad. Dermatol.* **2001**, *45*, 892–896. [CrossRef] [PubMed]
17. Lidstone, V.; Thorns, A. Pruritus in cancer patients. *Cancer Treat Rev.* **2001**, *27*, 305–312. [CrossRef]
18. Chiang, H.C.; Huang, V.; Cornelius, L.A. Cancer and itch. *Semin. Cutan. Med. Surg.* **2011**, *30*, 107–112. [CrossRef]
19. Jones, E.A.; Bergasa, N.V. Why do cholestatic patients itch? *Gut* **1996**, *38*, 644–645. [CrossRef]
20. Dawn, A.G.; Yosipovitch, G. Butorphanol for treatment of intractable pruritus. *J. Am. Acad. Dermatol.* **2006**, *54*, 527–531. [CrossRef]
21. Biggar, R.J.; Johansen, J.S.; Smedby, K.E.; Rostgaard, K.; Chang, E.T.; Adami, H.O.; Glimelius, B.; Molin, D.; Dutoit, S.H.; Melbye, M.; et al. Serum YKL-40 and interleukin 6 levels in Hodgkin lymphoma. *Clin. Cancer. Res.* **2008**, *14*, 6974–6978. [CrossRef] [PubMed]

22. Lee, H.L.; Eom, H.S.; Yun, T.; Kim, H.J.; Park, W.S.; Nam, B.H.; Moon-Wood, S.; Lee, D.H.; Kong, S.Y. Serum and urine levels of interleukin-8 in patients with non-Hodgkin's lymphoma. *Cytokine* **2008**, *43*, 71–75. [CrossRef] [PubMed]
23. Petrackova, M.; Hamsikova, E.; Duskova, M.; Ptackova, P.; Klamova, H.; Humlova, Z.; Vonka, V. Predictive value of serum cytokine levels in chronic myeloid leukemia patients. *Immunol. Lett.* **2016**, *179*, 61–67. [CrossRef] [PubMed]
24. Antosz, H.; Wojciechowska, K.; Sajewicz, J.; Choroszyńska, D.; Marzec-Kotarska, B.; Osiak, M.; Pajak, N.; Tomczak, W.; Baszak, M.J.; Baszakc, J. IL-6, IL-10, c-Jun and STAT3 expression in B-CLL. *Blood Cells Mol. Dis.* **2015**, *54*, 258–265. [CrossRef] [PubMed]

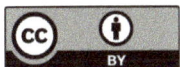

© 2019 by the authors. Licensee MDPI, Basel, Switzerland. This article is an open access article distributed under the terms and conditions of the Creative Commons Attribution (CC BY) license (http://creativecommons.org/licenses/by/4.0/).

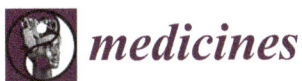

Article

Pruritus Associated with Commonly Prescribed Medications in a Tertiary Care Center

Amy H. Huang [1,2], Benjamin H. Kaffenberger [3], Adam Reich [4], Jacek C. Szepietowski [5], Sonja Ständer [6] and Shawn G. Kwatra [1,2,*]

1. Department of Dermatology, Johns Hopkins University School of Medicine, Baltimore, 21205 MD, USA
2. Bloomberg School of Public Health, Johns Hopkins University, Baltimore, 21205 MD, USA
3. Division of Dermatology, Ohio State University Wexner Medical Center, Columbus, 43210 OH, USA
4. Department of Dermatology, University of Rzeszow, 35-310 Rzeszow, Poland
5. Department of Dermatology, Venereology and Allergology, University of Medicine, 50-367 Wroclaw, Poland
6. Department of Dermatology, University Hospital of Münster, 48149 Münster, Germany
* Correspondence: skwatra1@jhmi.edu

Received: 16 July 2019; Accepted: 2 August 2019; Published: 4 August 2019

Abstract: Background: Sparse data are available on rates of drug-induced pruritus, a well-recognized adverse reaction. We sought to assess relative rates of pruritus associated with commonly prescribed medications. **Methods:** Using the electronic medical record system EPIC, retrospective data were collected on patients seen at Johns Hopkins who received a medication of interest in a five-year period (2013–2018). Sequential criteria were used to identify the subpopulation who presented with a chief complaint of "pruritus" or diagnosis of "itching" within three months of receiving drugs. **Results:** We identified 9802 patients with pruritus after drug initiation and 1,085,404 patients without. A higher proportion of those with pruritus were female (70%) than those without (58%), $p < 0.001$. Patients in both groups were most commonly 50 to 79 years old. A higher proportion of patients with pruritus were black (40%) compared to those without (23%), $p < 0.001$. In this study, the highest rates of pruritus were observed with heparin (1.11%), trimethoprim-sulfamethoxazole (1.06%), and calcium channel blockers (0.92%). Psychiatric/neurologic drugs used to treat pruritus were associated with low rates of itch. **Conclusions:** Certain cardiovascular and antimicrobial agents are associated with increased frequencies of pruritus. This knowledge may guide providers in clinical selection of commonly used agents to minimize adverse effects associated with reduced compliance.

Keywords: pruritus; itch; drug-induced; medication-related; epidemiology

1. Introduction

Drug-induced pruritus is a well-recognized adverse reaction, accounting for more than 10% of cutaneous drug reactions in previous studies [1]. Depending on the causative agent, symptoms may be acute in onset and resolve upon drug cessation or evolve into chronic pruritus lasting more than six weeks [1]. Skin lesions may or may not be visible as pruritus can result directly from inflammation of the skin or indirectly through systemic mediators, such as cholestatic liver injury [2,3]. In addition to negatively impacting quality of life, drug-induced pruritus has been associated with decreased medication compliance [4]. Despite this, sparse data are available on the association of pruritus with many commonly used medications. Previous studies have been limited to small case series or narrow in scope by focusing on a single healthcare setting or a single drug/drug class. In the present study, we use longitudinal data from an integrated health system to assess relative rates of pruritus associated with a variety of widely prescribed medications.

2. Materials and Methods

Institutional review board approval was waived because only anonymous aggregate-level data were used. Retrospective data on inpatient, outpatient, and emergency department (ED) visits were collected using the SlicerDicer feature of EPIC, the electronic medical record system of Johns Hopkins Health Systems (JHHS) [5]. The JHHS network includes tertiary care and community-based hospitals as well as a network of outpatient primary care/specialty clinics. In addition, a diverse patient population is served by the JHHS, due to the large local catchment area as well as domestic and international referrals for care.

2.1. Study Population

EPIC SlicerDicer was used to identify adult patients aged 18 years and older who were seen within JHHS within a five-year period (27 September 2013 to 27 September 2018) and received one or more medications of interest. Medications of interest were selected based on associations with pruritus in previous literature and frequency of usage in clinical practice [1–3]. Sequential criteria were used to specify the subpopulation who presented with a chief complaint of "pruritus" or diagnosis (visit or billing) of "itching" within three months of receiving medication, using the systematized nomenclature of medicine—clinical terms (SNOMED-CT). Chronic diagnoses of pruritus or itching were excluded to rule out other causes of itch unrelated to new medication. Three months was chosen as the time period of interest to allow for the expected delay between development of drug-induced pruritus and access to care where symptoms could be clinically documented. Among patients with pruritus, the SNOMED-CT term, "eruption of the skin", was used to identify those who developed an accompanying skin eruption in the same time period. "Eruption of the skin" is a parent term for most widespread skin diseases including rash, other nonspecific eruption of skin, and generalized drug eruption. The control population was comprised of adult patients aged 18 years and older seen in the same five-year period at JHHS who received a medication of interest, but without subsequent pruritus. Demographic variables including age, gender, and race were collected for both the study and control populations.

2.2. Medications of Interest

The three main drug classes queried were antimicrobial, cardiovascular, and psychiatric/neurologic drugs. For antimicrobials, numbers of patients developing subsequent pruritus with and without drug eruption were recorded for penicillin antibiotics, cephalosporins (first through fifth generation), macrolides, quinolones, tetracyclines, metronidazole, trimethoprim-sulfamethoxazole, and anti-malarial medications. For cardiovascular drugs, data was collected on angiotensin-converting enzyme (ACE) inhibitors, beta-blockers, calcium channel blockers, hydrochlorothiazide, amiodarone, heparin, and statins. For psychiatric/neurologic drugs, tricyclic antidepressants (TCAs), selective serotonin reuptake inhibitors (SSRIs), anti-epileptics, and opioid analgesics were investigated. Because of the smaller sample size of individual drugs, different drugs within the same category were grouped for increased power. For example, anti-epileptics were analyzed as an aggregate group and included carbamazepine, fosphenytoin, oxcarbazepine, phenytoin, and topiramate.

2.3. Statistical Analysis

Chi-squared tests were used to assess differences in proportions of categorical demographic variables (age, gender, and race) and rates of pruritus among different drug categories in Stata/IC15.1 (StataCorp, College Station, TX, USA). Pairwise student t-tests were also used to compare demographic variables, with a Bonferroni correction for multiple comparisons applied ($p < 0.003$ considered statistically significant). Frequencies of pruritus after receiving medication and of drug eruptions in those with pruritus were calculated using Microsoft Excel software (Microsoft Corporation, Redmond, WA, USA).

3. Results

3.1. Demographics

Of the patients studied, 9,802 developed pruritus, while 1,085,404 did not in the three-month period following initiation of the drug (Table 1). A higher proportion of patients with pruritus were female (70%) than those without (58%) ($p < 0.001$). Patients with pruritus were also more likely to be between 18–39 years of age compared to those without pruritus ($p < 0.001$). Patients in both groups were most commonly aged 50 to 79 years, but a greater percentage of patients with pruritus fell in this age group compared to those without, $p < 0.001$. A higher proportion of patients with pruritus were black (40%) as compared to patients without pruritus (23%), $p < 0.001$. In addition, a lower proportion of patients with pruritus were white or Native Hawaiian/Pacific Islander, respectively, compared to those without ($p < 0.001$, $p = 0.002$). Of the medications queried, the most commonly prescribed were opioid analgesics (n = 592,255), statins (n = 316,196), and cephalosporins (n = 252,342) (Table 2). The least commonly prescribed were amiodarone (n = 18,357), anti-epileptics (n = 38,147), and tricyclic anti-depressants (n = 38,147).

Table 1. Demographics.

Demographic	With Pruritus within 3 Months of Drug (n = 9802)	Without Pruritus After Receiving Drug (n = 1,085,404)	p-Value *	p-Value **
Gender, (%)				
Male	30.6	42.4	<0.001	<0.001
Female	69.4	57.6		<0.001
Age, (%)				
18–29	8.9	10.9		<0.001
30–39	11.8	13.8		<0.001
40–49	12.6	13.5		0.009
50–59	19.1	17.6		<0.001
60–69	20.4	18.8	<0.001	<0.001
70–79	16.3	14.8		<0.001
80–89	8.4	7.6		0.003
90–99	2.4	2.8		0.017
100+	0.1	0.2		0.027
Race (%)				
White/Caucasian	48.1	62.8		<0.001
Black/African American	38.9	23.1		<0.001
Asian	4.2	4.3		0.627
American Indian/Alaska Native	0.4	0.3	<0.001	0.072
Native Hawaiian/Pacific Islander	0.2	0.1		0.002
Other	7.7	7.4		0.259
Unknown	0.5	1.8		<0.001
Declined to answer	0.2	0.3		0.071

* Calculated by the chi-squared test for overall difference in proportions. ** Pairwise comparisons calculated using the student's *t*-test with Bonferroni correction for significance ($p < 0.003$).

Table 2. Total number of patients who received drugs during study period.

Drug Type	Number Who Received Drug (N)
Antimicrobial	
Penicillins	177,487
Cephalosporins	252,342
Macrolides	124,856
Quinolones	128,248
Tetracyclines	87,497
Metronidazole	66,074
TMP/SMX	73,579
Anti-malarials	80,949

Table 2. Cont.

Drug Type	Number Who Received Drug (N)
Cardiovascular	
ACEi	185,216
Beta-blockers	234,114
CCB	202,116
HCTZ	100,771
Amiodarone	18,357
Heparin	163,607
Statins	316,196
Psychiatric/Neurologic	
TCAs	43,756
SSRIs	212,244
Anti-epileptics	38,147
Opioid analgesics	592,255

3.2. Rates of Pruritus within Three Months of Receiving Drug

Rates of pruritus among drug classes queried were significantly different ($p < 0.001$). Among all drugs investigated, heparin (1.11%), trimethoprim–sulfamethoxazole (1.06%), and calcium channel blockers (0.92%) were associated with the highest rates of subsequent pruritus (Figure 1). In contrast, psychiatric/neurologic drugs as a class were associated with the lowest rates of subsequent pruritus: 0.1% in tricyclic anti-depressants, 0.03% in SSRIs, 0.05% in anti-epileptics, and 0.05% in opioid analgesics. Cardiovascular drugs were associated with generally higher rates of pruritus, with similar rates among ACE inhibitors (0.69%), beta-blockers (0.75%), hydrochlorothiazide (0.68%), amiodarone (0.62%), and statins (0.67%). Frequencies of subsequent pruritus were more varied among antimicrobial drugs. Higher rates of pruritus were associated with penicillin antibiotics (0.73%), macrolides (0.77%), and trimethoprim–sulfamethoxazole (1.06%) in contrast to relatively lower rates for cephalosporins (0.03%), quinolones (0.02%), tetracyclines (0.05%), metronidazole (0.04%), and anti-malarial drugs (0.01%).

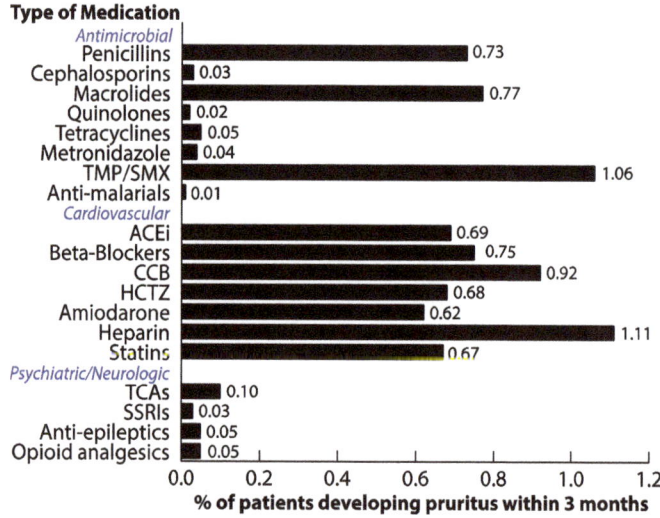

Figure 1. Frequency of pruritus after receiving drugs.

3.3. Rates of Drug Eruption among Patients with Pruritus Subsequent to Receiving Drug

In patients who developed pruritus, about half or fewer also developed skin eruption during the same time period (Figure 2). Rates of skin eruption in patients with pruritus were highest for cephalosporins (52.1%) and opioid analgesics (50.6%). Half (50.0%) of patients with pruritus who received quinolones and tetracyclines also developed skin eruptions, respectively. Rates of skin eruption among patients with pruritus after cardiovascular drugs were similar, ranging between 38.3% to 41.6% for all drugs queried. Frequencies of drug eruptions could not be reported for anti-malarial or anti-epileptic drugs, given the small absolute number of patients who experienced pruritus subsequent to initiation of these medications.

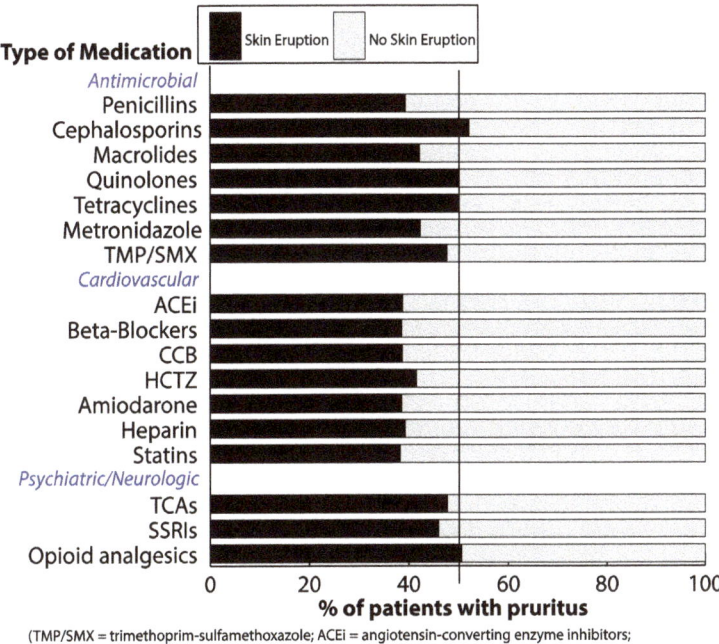

(TMP/SMX = trimethoprim-sulfamethoxazole; ACEi = angiotensin-converting enzyme inhibitors; CCB = calcium-channel blockers; HCTZ = hydrochlorothiazide; TCA = tricyclic antidepressants; SSRI = selective serotonin reuptake inhibitors)

Figure 2. Frequency of skin eruption in patients with pruritus after receiving drugs.

4. Discussion

Our findings confirm previous studies that have noted increased frequencies of drug-induced pruritus with certain antimicrobial and cardiovascular agents. Among antimicrobials, higher rates of pruritus with penicillin antibiotics and trimethoprim–sulfamethoxazole are thought to be secondary to inflammatory skin eruptions or cholestatic liver injury [1,3]. Among cardiovascular drugs, calcium channel blockers, beta blockers, and hydrochlorothiazide are associated with pruritus from skin inflammation, while itch with ACE inhibitors is thought to result from increased levels of bradykinin [3,6,7]. In addition, the rate of pruritus observed in statins (0.67%) is significant, considering its ubiquitous use as the second most commonly prescribed medication in the study (n = 316,196). Statin-induced xerosis cutis has been proposed as a potential mechanism of itch, with impaired barrier function resulting from decreased lipid distribution in the skin with inhibition of cholesterol biosynthesis [3]. In contrast, tricyclic antidepressants, SSRIs, and antiepileptics (including carbamazepine) were associated with low rates of pruritus. This is consistent with the established use of these agents to treat pruritus, through blockade of afferent neural pathways as well as direct action in the central nervous system [8].

Furthermore, we report that heparin was associated with a relatively high rate of pruritus (1.11%). This is in contrast to previous research noting rare heparin-induced itch primarily in the context of rare, IgE-mediated urticarial reactions [1]. The higher rate of heparin-induced pruritus in our study may capture a more frequent side effect of heparin: Pruritic, eczematous plaques at injection sites from delayed-type, non-IgE mediated allergic hypersensitivity (type IV) [9,10]. In contrast, we observed lower rates than previous studies of opioid-induced pruritus from triggering of non-immunological histamine release or effects on opioid receptors in the skin and central nervous system [11]. However, the frequency of opioid-induced pruritus is known to vary significantly—up to 50-fold—depending on the dosage, route of administration, and patient characteristics [12]. Lastly, macrolides have not been significantly implicated in previous literature of drug-related pruritus, but demonstrated a relatively high rate of subsequent pruritus in the present study (0.77%). Because of their significant anti-inflammatory properties, macrolides may have increased use in patients with chronic, inflammatory conditions that present episodically with pruritic flares [13]. It deserves further study whether macrolides also have the potential to invoke pruritus in individuals whose inflammatory condition may heighten their sensitivity to cutaneous side effects of medication [14].

To reduce confounding by indication, we compared relative rates of pruritus among patients who needed and received various drugs rather than to the healthier general population who did not. However, some residual confounding may remain as the drugs under study had a wide range of indications. Additional limitations of this study include its retrospective design and the use of aggregate data, which precluded multivariable analyses. Estimated rates of drug-induced pruritus may also be conservative and biased towards more severe reactions, given that cases were identified through clinical documentation of new itch with the Johns Hopkins Health System. Therefore, patients seen for drug-induced itch outside this network—such as at urgent care—may not be captured. Lastly, the small sample size of patients with pruritus limited our ability to perform specific subgroup analyses, despite evidence of ethnic differences in the development of itch (i.e., increased frequency with antimalarials in blacks) [15]. Furthermore, this also precluded analysis of demographics of patients with and without pruritus as stratified by inciting medication categories.

Of note, pre-existing pruritus in some patients improves upon initiation of antibiotics, but in this cohort, antibiotics were associated with subsequent pruritus [13]. Potential co-morbidities in these patients deserve further investigation, as tissue/nerve hypersensitivity in atopic or autoimmune conditions may contribute susceptibility to drug-induced pruritus [14]. We also observed a higher proportion of females in the group developing pruritus versus not (70% vs. 58%). This may be explained by pharmacokinetic and hormonal differences between genders that lead to differential drug metabolism, although their exact contribution to increased rates of adverse drug reactions in females is not well understood [16].

While overall rates of observed pruritus associated with medications were low (<1.2%), the relative frequency of pruritus with different medications within the same category (i.e., antimicrobials) varied up to 100-fold. Despite this significant magnitude of difference and the relatively higher rate of pruritus observed with certain medications, absolute correlation between these drugs and pruritus has not yet been proven. Future work in prospective studies should focus on elucidating drug-specific pathogenesis of itch to confirm these causal relationships. While difficult to quantify an exact threshold of pruritus frequency to establish high confidence of strong correlation between a certain drug and itch, the frequency threshold for clinical relevance is low. Given the high prevalence of these prescriptions in the patient population, even low absolute rates of drug-associated itch are clinically meaningful. Knowledge of relative rates of associated pruritus is therefore key to guiding provider selection of commonly used agents and minimizing adverse effects associated with reduced compliance.

Author Contributions: Conceptualization, A.H.H. and S.G.K.; Data curation, A.H.H.; Formal analysis, A.H.H.; Investigation, A.H.H. and S.G.K.; Methodology, A.H.H. and S.G.K.; Supervision, S.G.K.; Writing—Original draft, A.H.H. and S.G.K.; Writing—Review and editing, B.H.K., A.R., J.C.S., and S.S.

Funding: This research received no external funding.

Acknowledgments: Kwatra and Kaffenberger are recipients of the Dermatology Foundation Award. Kwatra is an advisory board member for Menlo and Trevi Therapeutics.

Conflicts of Interest: Dr. Kwatra is an advisory board member for Menlo and Trevi Therapeutics and has received grant funding from Kiniksa Pharmaceuticals. None of the other authors have any conflicts of interest to disclose.

References

1. Reich, A.; Stander, S.; Szepietowski, J.C. Drug-induced pruritus: A review. *Acta Derm. Venereol.* **2009**, *89*, 236–244. [CrossRef] [PubMed]
2. Peharda, V.; Gruber, F.; Kastelan, M.; Brajac, I.; Cabrijan, L. Pruritus an important symptom of internal diseases. *Acta Dermatoven. APA* **2000**, *9*, 92–104.
3. Garibyan, L.; Chiou, A.S.; Elmariah, S.B. Advanced aging skin and itch: Addressing an unmet need. *Dermatol. Ther.* **2013**, *26*, 92–103. [CrossRef] [PubMed]
4. Ajayi, A.A.; Kolawole, B.A.; Udoh, S.J. Endogenous opioids, μ-opiate receptors and chloroquine-induced pruritus: A double-blind comparison of naltrexone and promethazine in patients with malaria fever who have an established history of generalized chloroquine-induced itching. *Int. J. Dermatol.* **2004**, *43*, 972–977. [CrossRef] [PubMed]
5. Larson, V.A.; Tang, O.; Kang, S.; Kwatra, S.G. Association between itch and cancer in 16,925 patients with pruritus: Experience at a tertiary care center. *J. Am. Acad. Dermatol.* **2019**, *80*, 931–937. [CrossRef] [PubMed]
6. Summers, E.M.; Bingham, C.S.; Dahle, K.W.; Sweeney, C.; Ying, J.; Sontheimer, R.D. Chronic eczematous eruptions in the aging: Further support for an association with exposure to calcium channel blockers. *JAMA Dermatol.* **2013**, *149*, 814–818. [CrossRef] [PubMed]
7. Steckelings, U.; Artuc, M.; Wollschlager, T.; Wiehstutz, S.; Henz, B. Angiotensin-converting enzyme inhibitors as inducers of adverse cutaneous reactions. *Acta Derm. Venereol.* **2001**, *81*, 321–325. [CrossRef] [PubMed]
8. Steinhoff, M.; Cevikbas, F.; Ikoma, A.; Berger, T.G. Pruritus: Management algorithms and experimental therapies. *Semin. Cutan. Med. Surg.* **2011**, *30*, 127–137. [CrossRef] [PubMed]
9. Schindewolf, M.; Schwaner, S.; Wolter, M.; Kroll, H.; Recke, A.; Kaufmann, R.; Boehncke, W.H.; Lindhoff-Last, E.; Ludwig, R.J. Incidence and causes of heparin-induced skin lesions. *Can. Med. Assoc. J.* **2009**, *181*, 477–481. [CrossRef] [PubMed]
10. Trautmann, A.; Seitz, C.S. Heparin allergy: Delayed-type non-ige-mediated allergic hypersensitivity to subcutaneous heparin injection. *Immunol. Allergy Clin. N. Am.* **2009**, *29*, 469–480. [CrossRef] [PubMed]
11. Waxler, B.; Dadabhoy, Z.P.; Stojiljkovic, L.; Rabito, S.F. Primer of Postoperative pruritus for anesthesiologists. *Anesthesiology* **2005**, *103*, 168–178. [CrossRef] [PubMed]
12. Reich, A.; Szepietowski, J.C. Opioid-induced pruritus: an update. *Clin. Exp. Dermatol.* **2009**, *35*, 2–6. [CrossRef] [PubMed]
13. Alzolibani, A.A.; Zedan, K. Macrolides in chronic inflammatory skin disorders. *Mediat. Inflamm.* **2012**, 1–7. [CrossRef] [PubMed]
14. Luo, J.; Feng, J.; Liu, S.; Walters, E.T.; Hu, H. Molecular and cellular mechanisms that initiate pain and itch. *Cell Mol. Life Sci.* **2015**, *72*, 3201–3223. [CrossRef] [PubMed]
15. Ajayi, A.A.L. Itching, chloroquine, and malaria: A review of recent molecular and neuroscience advances and their contribution to mechanistic understanding and therapeutics of chronic non-histaminergic pruritus. *Int. J. Dermatol.* **2019**, *58*, 880–891. [CrossRef] [PubMed]
16. Rademaker, M. Do women have more adverse drug reactions? *Am. J. Clin. Dermatol.* **2001**, *2*, 349–351. [CrossRef] [PubMed]

© 2019 by the authors. Licensee MDPI, Basel, Switzerland. This article is an open access article distributed under the terms and conditions of the Creative Commons Attribution (CC BY) license (http://creativecommons.org/licenses/by/4.0/).

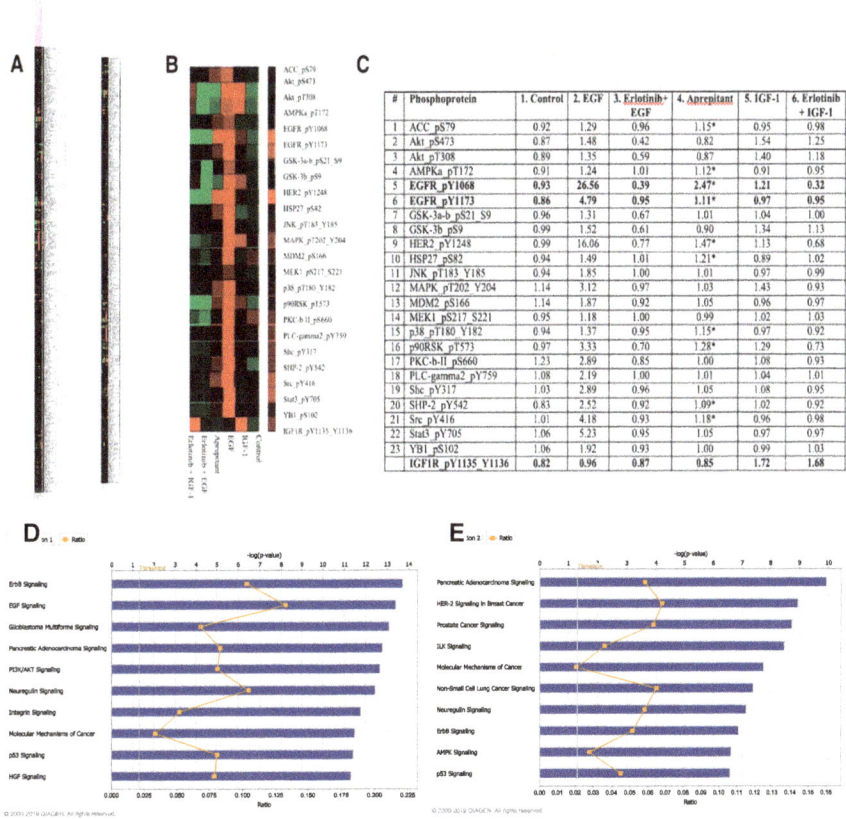

Figure 1. Proteomic analysis of HaCaT cells using reverse phase protein array (RPPA) technology. (**A**) Unsupervised and supervised heatmaps from RPPA analysis on HaCaT cells treated with the following agents: Control (DMSO only), EGF (100 ng/mL) for 10 min, IGF-1 (100 ng/mL) for 10 min, erlotinib (10 µM) for 60 min followed by EGF (100 ng/mL) for 10 min, erlotinib (10 µM) for 60 min followed by IGF-1 (100 ng/mL) for 10 min, aprepitant (10 µM) for 60 min. (**B**) A section of heatmap focusing on intracellular proteins phosphorylated by epidermal growth factor receptor (EGFR) activation. (**C**) List of 23 phosphoproteins whose phosphorylation increased by more than 20% upon stimulation of EGFR by EGF. Phosphorylation of 10 of these proteins (43% of the total phosphorylated upon EGF stimulation) also increased following treatment with aprepitant (marked with an asterisk). (**D**) Top 10 pathways determined by Ingenuity Pathway Analysis of RPPA data from control and EGF-stimulated HaCaT cells. (**E**). Top 10 pathways determined by Ingenuity Pathway Analysis of RPPA data from control and aprepitant-treated HaCaT cells.

3. Results

Figure 1A show shows the results of RPPA analysis on HaCaT cell lysates treated with the following conditions: Control, EGF, IGF-1, erlotinib followed by EGF, erlotinib followed by IGF-1, and aprepitant. Figure 1B shows the RPPA analysis results with a focus on the intracellular proteins that were phosphorylated by EGFR activation. Figure 1C lists the HaCaT human keratinocyte proteins whose phosphorylation increased by at least 20% upon stimulation by EGF. The EGF-induced increase in the phosphorylation of these proteins (Figure 1C, column 2) was mediated through EGFR, because no increase in phosphorylation was seen with EGF when the cells were pre-treated with the EGFR-tyrosine of RPPA lysis buffer (1% Triton X-100, 50 mM 4-(2-hydroxyethyl)-1-piperazineethanesulfonic acid (HEPES) pH 7.4, 150 mM NaCl, 1.5 mM $MgCl_2$, 1 mM egtazic acid (EGTA), 100 mM NaF, 10 mM Na pyrophosphate, 1 mM Na_3VO_4, 10% glycerol, plus a cocktail of protease and phosphatase inhibitors (recipe provided by M.D. Anderson's Reverse Phase Protein Array core facility)), centrifuged, and processed according to the instructions provided by the RPPA core facility [15].

2.2. Ingenuity Pathway Analysis of RPPA Data

Ingenuity pathway analysis (IPA) suite (Qiagen, Germany) was separately run on RPPA data from cells treated with EGF and aprepitant. The top ten canonical pathways affected (ranked by p value from Fisher's exact test) by these treatments were determined. The "threshold" (vertical dotted line) shows a p value of 0.05. The "ratio" (line with points on each bar) refers to the proportion of molecules in the dataset that mapped to IPA's canonical pathway.

2.3. Western Blotting

Changes in EGFR phosphorylation in HaCaT cells and NHEK primary keratinocytes were visualized using Western blotting (Figure 1A–D) as described previously [15]. Briefly, approximately 500,000 freshly dissociated HaCaT or primary keratinocytes were plated in six-well plates containing 5 mL of media. After 24 h, the media was changed to 5 mL of serum-free media and cells were incubated for one hour with dimethylsulfoxide (DMSO) (control and EGF groups) or with different concentrations of aprepitant in DMSO in a 37 °C, 5% CO_2 incubator. After this incubation, the cells in one well (EGF group) were treated with 5 µL of 100 µg/mL EGF for 10 min. The media was removed from all wells and cells were washed twice with ice-cold PBS. The washed cell pellets were added to 100 µL of RPPA lysis buffer and the protein concentration was measured, as detailed previously [15]. About 10 µg of lysate proteins from each treatment group was run on a 4–12% NovexBis-Tris gel (Life Technologies, Grand Island, NY, USA). The separated proteins were transferred to a polyvinylidene difluoride membrane, blocked with 5% milk, then probed with a rabbit polyclonal p-EGFR Y1068 antibody (catalog #2234; Cell Signaling Technology, Beverly, MA, USA) or a rabbit polyclonal EGFR antibody to detect total EGFR. Rabbit Beta-Actin antibody was used to show equal protein loading. The blot was developed using the Pierce Enhanced Chemiluminescence (ECL) Western Blotting Substrate Kit (cat #32106, ThermoFisher Scientific, Waltham, MA, USA) and Biomax MR film (Sigma-Aldrich Corp., St. Louis, MO, USA).

2.4. Effect of EGF and Aprepitant on the Growth of HaCaT Cells

The effect of EGF and aprepitant on the growth of HaCaT cells was determined using the WST-1 Cell Proliferation Assay System according to the manufacturer's instructions (cat #MK400Takara Bio USA; Mountainview, CA). Briefly, freshly dissociated HaCaT cells were seeded in a 96-well plate at a density of 2000–5000 cells/well in 200 µL of media. The plates were placed in a cell culture incubator (37 °C, 5% CO_2) overnight and the media was changed to serum-free media. After 24 h, cells were treated with different concentrations of EGF (dissolved in PBS) and aprepitant (dissolved in DMSO). Each concentration of EGF and aprepitant was tested in quadruplicate. After incubating the cells for 3–4 days in the incubator, 20 µL of WST-1 reagent was added to each well. The cells were again incubated in the incubator for 1–4 h, and absorbance was measured at a wavelength of 450 nm using Biorad's Bench Mark Plus plate reader (Hercules, CA, USA). Background absorbance was measured by adding the WST-1 reagent to wells containing the media but no cells. The experiment was repeated four times and the data were analyzed using GraphPad Prism 5.0 software (San Diego, CA, USA).

by genetic ablation of epidermal EGFR in a mouse model [4]. Similarly, a loss-of-function mutation of EGFR in a human child exhibited skin toxicity resembling that seen in patients taking EGFR inhibitors [5].

The effects of erlotinib-induced pruritus on quality of life is substantial; 12–16% of all cancer patients treated with erlotinib develop pruritus, usually within the first few days to weeks of therapy [6]. In addition to its significant effect on psychosocial well-being, pruritus can also interfere with treatment efficacy by leading to poor drug compliance and even dose modifications or discontinuation by healthcare providers [1,7]. A survey of oncologists from 2010 revealed that 76% of practitioners modified a patient's dose of EGFR inhibitors in response to the associated skin toxicities, and 32% discontinued EGFR inhibitor therapy altogether [8]. Thus, understanding and preventing EGFR inhibitor skin toxicity is critical to improving patient quality of life and survival.

In recent years, neurokinin-1 receptor (NK1R) antagonists such as aprepitant have emerged as a promising class of medications for the treatment of chronic pruritus [9]. In 2009, a case series in the New England Journal of Medicine first described the successful off-label use of aprepitant to treat severe, recalcitrant itch in three patients with cutaneous T-cell lymphoma (CTCL) [10]. Since then, a case series of cancer patients showed prompt relief of erlotinib-induced itch after administration of aprepitant [11]. Furthermore, a clinical trial in 2012 established the efficacy of aprepitant in reducing pruritus caused by anti-EGFR therapy [12]. The current proposed mechanism for aprepitant's antipruritic effect is the prevention of the neuropeptide substance P (SP) from binding to NK1R on the surface of dermal mast cells, thus preventing mast cell activation and degranulation [13]. However, this theory remains unconfirmed, and the effect of aprepitant on human keratinocytes remains largely unexplored.

To better understand the effect of aprepitant on human keratinocytes, we examined the effects of aprepitant on EGFR signaling in HaCaT cells—an immortalized line of human keratinocytes [14]—using reverse phase protein array (RPPA) technology.

2. Materials and Methods

Human HaCaT keratinocytes cells were obtained from Dr. Xiao-Fan Wang, Duke University, and were cultured in Dulbecco's modified Eagle's medium (DMEM) (Gibco Cat #11960-044), supplemented with 10% fetal bovine serum (FBS) (Sigma, cat #F2442) and 1% L-glutamine (Ionza, cat #17-605E). The HaCaT cell line was authenticated by short tandem repeat (STR) DNA profiling using the Promega GenePrint 10 kit (Promega Cat #B9510) by the Duke University DNA Analysis Facility. The observed STR profile was Amelogenin: (X,Y); CSF1PO: (11,11); D13S317: (11,12); D16S539: (9,9); D5S818: (12,12); D7S820: (9,11); TH01: (9.3,9.3); TPOX: (8,12); vWA: (15,15); D21S11: (28,29). Normal Human Epidermal Keratinocytes (NHEK), isolated from the skin of a 23-year-old female, were purchased from PromoCell GmbH, Heidelberg, Germany (cat #C-12003; lot #401Z028.1). These cells were grown in the media provided by the manufacturer. Primary antibodies to detect total EGFR (cat #2232), EGFR-pY1068 (cat #2234), goat anti-rabbit (cat #7074), and anti-biotin (cat #7075) were purchased from Cell Signaling Technology. Aprepitant was purchased from APExBIO, Houston, TX (cat #A1684). Substance P and epidermal growth factor (EGF) were obtained from Sigma (St. Louis, MO). Human insulin-like growth factor-1 (IGF-1) was purchased from Gibco/ThermoFisher (cat #PHG0078). Erlotinib hydrochloride (cat #E-4007) was purchased from LC laboratories (Woburn, MA, USA).

2.1. Preparation of HaCaT Cells for RPPA Analysis

HaCaT cells (5×10^5) were placed in each well of a six-well plate. The next day, the medium was changed to serum-free. After 24 h in serum-free media, the cells were treated with various drugs. To examine the stimulation of EGFR by EGF, the cells were treated with EGF (100 ng/mL) for 10 min. To examine the blockade of EGF stimulation of EGFR by erlotinib, the cells were treated with erlotinib for 1 h followed by 10 min of exposure to EGF. To study the stimulation of EGFR with aprepitant and other NK1R blockers, cells were treated with these drugs for 1 h. After the treatment, the media was removed and the cells were washed twice with ice-cold PBS. The washed cells were taken in 120 μL

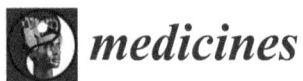

Article

Proteomic and Phosphoproteomic Analysis Reveals that Neurokinin-1 Receptor (NK1R) Blockade with Aprepitant in Human Keratinocytes Activates a Distinct Subdomain of EGFR Signaling: Implications for the Anti-Pruritic Activity of NK1R Antagonists

Shawn G. Kwatra [1], Emily Boozalis [1], Amy H. Huang [1], Cory Nanni [2], Raveena Khanna [1], Kyle A. Williams [1], Yevgeniy R. Semenov [3], Callie M. Roberts [2], Robert F. Burns [2], Madison Krischak [2] and Madan M. Kwatra [2,4,*]

[1] Department of Dermatology, Johns Hopkins University, Baltimore, MD 21287, USA; skwatra1@jhmi.edu (S.G.K.); eboozalis@gmail.com (E.B.); ahuang32@jhmi.edu (A.H.H.); rkhanna8@jhmi.edu (R.K.); kwill184@health.fau.edu (K.A.W.)
[2] Department of Anesthesiology, Duke University, Durham, NC 27710, USA; cory.nanni@duke.edu (C.N.); callie.roberts@duke.edu (C.M.R.); robert.burns@duke.edu (R.F.B.); madison.krischak@duke.edu (M.K.)
[3] Division of Dermatology, Washington University School of Medicine, St. Louis, MI 63110, USA; yevgeniy.semenov1@gmail.com
[4] Department of Pharmacology and Cancer Biology, Duke University Medical Center, Durham, NC 27710, USA
* Correspondence: madan.kwatra@duke.edu

Received: 10 September 2019; Accepted: 11 November 2019; Published: 9 December 2019

Abstract: Background: Epidermal growth factor receptor (EGFR) inhibitors can cause serious cutaneous toxicities, including pruritus and papulopustular acneiform skin eruptions. Increasingly, the neurokinin-1 receptor (NK1R) antagonist aprepitant is being utilized as an anti-pruritic agent in the treatment of EGFR-inhibitor induced pruritus. Aprepitant is believed to reduce itching by blocking NK1R on the surface of dermal mast cells. However, the effects of aprepitant on human keratinocytes remains unexplored. **Methods**: Herein, we examine the effects of aprepitant on EGFR stimulation in HaCaT cells using a phosphoproteomic approach including reverse phase protein arrays and Ingenuity Pathway Analysis. Changes in EGFR phosphorylation were visualized using Western blotting and the effect of EGF and aprepitant on the growth of HaCaT cells was determined using the WST-1 Cell Proliferation Assay System. **Results**: We found that aprepitant increased the phosphorylation of EGFR, as well as 10 of the 23 intracellular proteins phosphorylated by EGF. Analysis of phosphoproteomic data using Ingenuity Pathway Analysis software revealed that 5 of the top 10 pathways activated by EGF and aprepitant are shared. **Conclusions**: We propose that aprepitant produces its antipruritic effects by partially activating EGFR. Activation of EGFR by aprepitant was also seen in primary human keratinocytes. In addition to itch reduction through partial activation of shared EGFR pathways, aprepitant exerts a dose-dependent cytotoxicity to epithelial cells, which may contribute to its antitumor effects.

Keywords: aprepitant; erlotinib; pruritus; EGFR; epidermal growth factor receptor; NK1R; neurokinin1-receptor

1. Introduction

Epidermal growth factor receptor (EGFR) inhibitors such as erlotinib can cause serious cutaneous toxicities, including papulopustular acneiform skin eruptions and severe pruritus [1–3]. The skin toxicity of EGFR inhibitors is due to the blockade of EGFR in the epidermis, which was demonstrated kinase inhibitor (TKI) erlotinib (Figure 1C, column 3). Figure 1C, column 4 shows HaCaT cell proteins whose phosphorylation was increased when exposed to aprepitant. Proteins marked with an asterisk demonstrated an increase in phosphorylation. As can be seen, 10 out of 23 proteins phosphorylated by EGF stimulation were also phosphorylated by aprepitant, albeit not as robustly as EGF. These data indicate that aprepitant in HaCaT cells serves as a partial agonist of EGFR. Interestingly, cross-talk between EGFR and NK1R was also reported in human mesenteric preadipocytes, but in these cells EGFR phosphorylation was increased by substance P (SP), an agonist of NK1R [16]. There are additional examples of SP increasing the phosphorylation of EGFR [17,18]. However, none of these reports came from keratinocytes. To our knowledge, the keratinocyte is the only cell type where EGFR phosphorylation is increased by an NK1R antagonist. The mechanism by which NK1R blockade, rather than stimulation, in keratinocytes increases EGFR phosphorylation remains to be determined. However, our preliminary data indicate that keratinocytes express only the truncated isoform of NK1R (Kwatra et al., unpublished data).

We also treated HaCaT cells with IGF-1, because IGF-1 was implicated in the transmodulation of EGFR in keratinocytes [19]. As expected, IGF-1 stimulation of HaCaT cells increased the phosphorylation of IGF-1R at Y1135 and Y1137 (last row in Figure 1C) indicating that IGF-1R in HaCaT cells was functional. IGF-1 also increased the phosphorylation of EGFR (visualized in columns 1 and 5). Further, IGF-1 increased the phosphorylation of p90RSK_T543, which was blocked by erlotinib. Thus, our data showed that a downstream kinase of EGFR signaling was activated by IGF-1 and was blocked by erlotinib. Taken together, our results provide direct evidence of IGF-1 activation of EGFR in keratinocytes, which was suggested by previous reports [16]. However, the increase in EGFR signaling by IGF-1 was much less than that seen with aprepitant (compare columns 4 and 5).

To obtain further insight into aprepitant's mechanism of action, Ingenuity Pathway Analysis software was used to compare the top ten pathways activated by EGF (Figure 1D) and aprepitant (Figure 1E). These data show that five of the top ten signaling pathways activated by EGF and aprepitant are shared: ErbB, Pancreatic Adenocarcinoma, Neuregulin, Molecular Mechanisms of Cancer, and p53.

To confirm the observed aprepitant-induced increase in EGFR phosphorylation seen with RPPA analysis (Figure 1C), Western blotting was utilized (Figure 2). As Figure 2A shows, aprepitant increased the phosphorylation of EGFR in a dose-dependent manner. Note that the antibody that was used for total EGFR (catalog #2232, Cell Signaling Technology, Danvers, MA, USA) was raised against a peptide from an EGFR sequence that included Y1068; therefore, it did not recognize EGFR when it was phosphorylated at Y1068 (this explains why we had a weaker band for total EGFR when the receptor was phosphorylated).

We next examined whether aprepitant-induced EGFR activation seen in HaCaT cells, a cell line derived from human keratinocytes, was also seen in primary human keratinocytes (NHEK) cells. As Figure 2B shows, aprepitant also stimulated the phosphorylation of EGFR in NHEK cells in a dose-dependent manner.

Finally, the effects of aprepitant on cell division, as measured by the WST-1 Cell Proliferation Assay, were tested by incubating HaCaT cells with different concentrations of aprepitant and EGF, respectively. As expected, HaCaT cells demonstrated a significant dose-dependent increase in cell proliferation upon incubation with EGF as compared to PBS (Figure 3A). In contrast, HaCaT cells showed a significant dose-dependent cell death with increasing concentrations of aprepitant (Figure 3B).

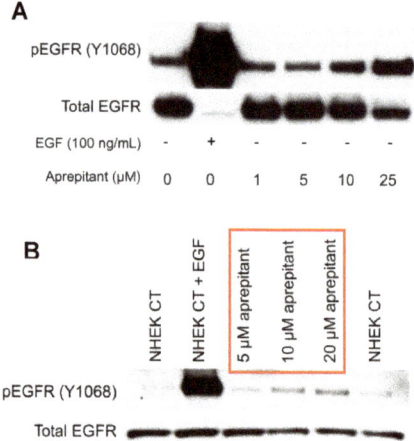

Figure 2. Visualization of EGFR phosphorylation at Y1068 by Western blotting. (**A**) HaCaT cells were treated with different concentrations of aprepitant. Western blot analysis showed that aprepitant stimulated the phosphorylation of EGFR in a dose-dependent manner. (**B**) Normal Human Epidermal Keratinocytes (NHEK) cells were treated with different concentrations of aprepitant. Western blot analysis showed that aprepitant increased the phosphorylation of EGFR in primary keratinocytes in a dose-dependent manner, similar to that seen in HaCaT cells.

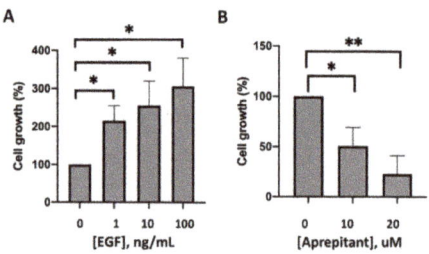

Figure 3. Effects of EGF and aprepitant on growth of HaCaT Cells. (**A**) HaCaT cells treated with EGF showed a significant dose-dependent increase in cell proliferation compared to incubation with PBS alone. (**B**) HaCaT cells treated with aprepitant (AP) showed a significant dose-dependent significant increase in cell death compared to incubation with DMSO alone. (* indicates $p < 0.05$, ** indicates $p < 0.01$).

4. Discussion

A key finding of our study was that aprepitant activated EGFR in human keratinocytes, a novel finding that may explain aprepitant's anti-pruritic activity. Despite partial activation of EGFR in keratinocytes, aprepitant also demonstrated dose-dependent cytotoxicity to epithelial cells in our study that was consistent with previous reports of its anti-tumor effects [20–22]. One hypothesis for this phenomenon is that the truncated form of NK1R may predominate in human skin, in addition to being overexpressed in tumor cells. In contrast, the full-length form of NK1R is typically expressed in normal non-tumor cells. This difference may explain the dose-dependent toxicity of aprepitant that was observed in HaCaT cells. It should be noted, however, that aprepitant-induced cytotoxicity should be negligible at doses lower than 10 μM that are used for anti-pruritic effects.

The cutaneous reactions seen in erlotinib-treated patients appear to be clinical indicators of treatment response, with the severity of cutaneous toxicities also appearing to be dose-dependent [6,23]. There is also a strong positive correlation between the severity of cutaneous toxicity following EGFR inhibition and overall patient survival [24]. Thus, despite the adverse effects on quality of life and compliance, the presence of cutaneous symptoms in these cancer patients may be viewed as a positive event. Therefore, aprepitant may be recommended as a therapeutic option for management of EGFR-TKI-induced itch [4].

The pathophysiology of tyrosine-kinase inhibitor-induced pruritus is incompletely understood, and data studying this phenomenon are sparse [23]. It is important to understand the mechanism underlying EGFR inhibitor-induced pruritus and skin toxicity to prevent premature termination of chemotherapy and to improve quality of life in cancer patients. Future studies should be directed at further understanding the mechanism of EGFR-TKI-induced pruritus and skin toxicity in order to better develop pharmacotherapies to relieve symptoms without interfering with cancer treatment.

In summary, our findings demonstrated that aprepitant activated EGFR in human keratinocytes by interacting with NK1R, and this might be the mechanism by which aprepitant reduces erlotinib-induced pruritus and skin toxicity.

We also showed that, in addition to partial activation of EGFR that may mediate its antipruritic effects, aprepitant also displayed antitumoral effects in suppressing cell growth. Future research on EGFR signaling and skin cytotoxicity in patients receiving the U.S. Food and Drug Administration (FDA)-approved doses of aprepitant is needed to verify the effects of aprepitant on human keratinocytes in vivo.

Author Contributions: Conceptualization, S.G.K., M.K., and M.M.K.; data curation, S.G.K., A.H.H., C.N., Y.R.S., C.M.R., R.F.B., M.K., and M.M.K.; formal analysis, A.H.H., Y.R.S., and M.M.K.; investigation, A.H.H., C.N., Y.R.S., C.M.R., R.F.B., and M.K.; methodology, A.H.H., C.N., Y.R.S., C.M.R., R.F.B., M.K., and M.M.K.; project administration, M.K. and M.M.K.; resources, M.M.K.; software, A.H.H.; supervision, M.K. and M.M.K.; validation, Y.R.S.; writing—original draft, E.B. and R.K.; writing—review and editing, S.G.K., A.H.H., R.K., K.A.W., M.K., and M.M.K.

Funding: Shawn Kwatra is a recipient of the Dermatology Foundation's Medical Dermatology Career Development Award. Madan Kwatra is funded by NIH grant #R21NS078642.

Conflicts of Interest: Shawn G. Kwatra is an advisory board member for Trevi and Menlo therapeutics and has received grant funding from Kiniska Pharmaceuticals. The other authors have no conflicts of interest to declare. The funders had no role in the design of the study; in the collection, analyses, or interpretation of data; in the writing of the manuscript, or in the decision to publish the results.

References

1. Lacouture, M.E.; Anadkat, M.J.; Bensadoun, R.J.; Bryce, J.; Chan, A.; Epstein, J.B.; Eaby-Sandy, B.; Murphy, B.A. Clinical practice guidelines for the prevention and treatment of EGFR inhibitor-associated dermatologic toxicities. *Support. Care Cancer* **2011**, *19*, 1079–1095. [CrossRef] [PubMed]
2. Kang, H.J.; Loftus, S.; Taylor, A.; DiCristina, C.; Green, S.; Zwaan, C.M. Aprepitant for the prevention of chemotherapy-induced nausea and vomiting in children: A randomised, double-blind, phase 3 trial. *Lancet Oncol.* **2015**, *16*, 385–394. [CrossRef]
3. Kaul, S.; Kaffenberger, B.H.; Choi, J.N.; Kwatra, S.G. Cutaneous Adverse Reactions of Anticancer Agents. *Dermatol. Clin.* **2019**, *37*, 555–568. [CrossRef] [PubMed]
4. Mascia, F.; Lam, G.; Keith, C.; Garber, C.; Steinberg, S.M.; Kohn, E.; Yuspa, S.H. Genetic Ablation of Epidermal EGFR Reveals the Dynamic Origin of Adverse Effects of Anti-EGFR Therapy. *Sci. Transl. Med.* **2013**, *5*, 199ra110. [CrossRef]
5. Campbell, P.; Morton, P.E.; Takeichi, T.; Salam, A.; Roberts, N.; Proudfoot, L.E.; Mellerio, J.E.; Aminu, K.; Wellington, C.; Patil, S.N.; et al. Epithelial Inflammation Resulting from an Inherited Loss-of-Function Mutation in EGFR. *J. Investig. Dermatol.* **2014**, *134*, 2570–2578. [CrossRef]
6. Lichtenberger, B.M.; Gerber, P.A.; Holcmann, M.; Buhren, B.A.; Amberg, N.; Smolle, V.; Schrumpf, H.; Boelke, E.; Ansari, P.; Mackenzie, C.; et al. Epidermal EGFR Controls Cutaneous Host Defense and Prevents Inflammation. *Sci. Transl. Med.* **2013**, *5*, 199ra111. [CrossRef]
7. Larson, V.A.; Tang, O.; Stander, S.; Kang, S.; Kwatra, S.G. Association between itch and cancer in 16,925 patients with pruritus: Experience at a tertiary care center. *J. Am. Acad. Dermatol.* **2019**, *80*, 931–937. [CrossRef]

8. Hassel, J.C.; Kripp, M.; Al-Batran, S.; Hofheinz, R.-D. Treatment of Epidermal Growth Factor Receptor Antagonist-Induced Skin Rash: Results of a Survey among German Oncologists. *Oncol. Res. Treat.* **2010**, *33*, 94–98. [CrossRef]
9. He, A.; Alhariri, J.M.; Sweren, R.J.; Kwatra, M.M.; Kwatra, S.G. Aprepitant for the Treatment of Chronic Refractory Pruritus. *Biomed. Res. Int.* **2017**, *2017*. [CrossRef]
10. Duval, A.; Dubertret, L. Aprepitant as an Antipruritic Agent? *N. Engl. J. Med.* **2009**, *361*, 1415–1416. [CrossRef]
11. Vincenzi, B.; Tonini, G.; Santini, D. Aprepitant for Erlotinib-Induced Pruritus. *N. Engl. J. Med.* **2010**, *363*, 397–398. [CrossRef] [PubMed]
12. Santini, D.; Vincenzi, B.; Guida, F.M.; Imperatori, M.; Schiavon, G.; Venditti, O.; Frezza, A.M.; Berti, P.; Tonini, G. Aprepitant for management of severe pruritus related to biological cancer treatments: A pilot study. *Lancet Oncol.* **2012**, *13*, 1020–1024. [CrossRef]
13. Gerber, P.A.; Buhren, B.A.; Homey, B. More on Aprepitant for Erlotinib-Induced Pruritus. *N. Engl. J. Med.* **2011**, *364*, 486–487. [PubMed]
14. Marqués, M.M.; Martínez, N.; Rodríguez-García, I.; Alonso, A. EGFR Family-Mediated Signal Transduction in the Human Keratinocyte Cell Line HaCaT. *Exp. Cell Res.* **1999**, *252*, 432–438. [CrossRef] [PubMed]
15. Brown, K.E.; Chagoya, G.; Kwatra, S.G.; Yen, T.; Keir, S.T.; Cooter, M.; Hoadley, K.A.; Rasheed, A.; Lipp, E.S.; Mclendon, R.; et al. Proteomic profiling of patient-derived glioblastoma xenografts identifies a subset with activated EGFR: Implications for drug development. *J. Neurochem.* **2015**, *133*, 730–738. [CrossRef]
16. Gross, K.; Karagiannides, I.; Thomou, T.; Koon, H.W.; Bowe, C.; Kim, H.; Giorgadze, N.; Tchkonia, T.; Pirtskhalava, T.; Kirkland, J.L.; et al. Substance P promotes expansion of human mesenteric preadipocytes through proliferative and antiapoptotic pathways. *Am. J. Physiol. Gastrointest. Liver Physiol.* **2009**, *296*, G1012–G1019. [CrossRef]
17. Castagliuolo, I.; Valenick, L.; Liu, J.; Pothoulakis, C. Epidermal growth factor receptor transactivation mediates substance P-induced mitogenic responses in U-373 MG cells. *J. Biol. Chem.* **2000**, *275*, 26545–26550. [CrossRef]
18. Wang, J.G.; Yu, J.; Hu, J.L.; Yang, W.L.; Ren, H.; Ding, D.; Zhang, L.; Liu, X.P. Neurokinin-1 activation affects EGFR-related signal transduction in triple ngetaive breast cancer. *Cell Signal.* **2015**, *27*, 1315–1324. [CrossRef]
19. Ando, Y.; Jensen, P.J. Epidermal Growth Factor and Insulin-Like Growth Factor I Enhance Keratinocyte Migration. *J. Investig. Dermatol.* **1993**, *100*, 633–639. [CrossRef]
20. Munoz, M.; Rosso, M. The NK-1 receptor antagonist aprepitant as a broad spectrum antitumor drug. *Investig. New Drugs* **2010**, *28*, 187–193. [CrossRef]
21. Muñoz, M.; Rosso, M.; Robles-Frias, M.J.; Salinas-Martín, M.V.; Rosso, R.; González-Ortega, A.; Coveñas, R. The NK-1 receptor is expressed in human melanoma and is involved in the antitumor action of the NK-1 receptor antagonist aprepitant on melanoma cell lines. *Lab Investig.* **2010**, *90*, 1259–1269. [CrossRef]
22. Kwatra, S.G.; Boozalis, E.; Kwatra, M.M. Effects of neuroimmune axis modulation by aprepitant on antipruritic and global disease severity in patients with cutaneous T-cell lymphoma. *Br. J. Dermatol.* **2018**, *178*, 1221–1222. [CrossRef] [PubMed]
23. Lacouture, M.E.; Rodeck, U. Skinflammation and Drug Toxicity—A Delicate Balance. *Sci. Transl. Med.* **2013**, *5*, 199fs33. [CrossRef] [PubMed]
24. Chanprapaph, K.; Vachiramon, V.; Rattanakaemakorn, P. Epidermal Growth Factor Receptor Inhibitors: A Review of Cutaneous Adverse Events and Management. *Dermatol. Res. Pract.* **2014**, *2014*, 734249. [CrossRef] [PubMed]

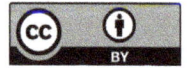 © 2019 by the authors. Licensee MDPI, Basel, Switzerland. This article is an open access article distributed under the terms and conditions of the Creative Commons Attribution (CC BY) license (http://creativecommons.org/licenses/by/4.0/).

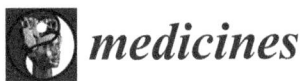

Article

Role of Dysregulated Ion Channels in Sensory Neurons in Chronic Kidney Disease-Associated Pruritus

Akishi Momose [1,*], Micihihiro Yabe [1], Shigetoshi Chiba [1], Kenjirou Kumakawa [1], Yasuo Shiraiwa [1] and Hiroki Mizukami [2]

1. Department of Urology, Jusendo General Hospital, Koriyama 9638585, Japan; m.yabe@jusendo.or.jp (M.Y.); s.chiba@jusendo.or.jp (S.C.); k.kumakawa@jusendo.or.jp (K.K.); y.shiraiwa@jusendo.or.jp (Y.S.)
2. Department of Pathology and Molecular Medicine, Hirosaki University Graduate School of Medicine, Hirosaki 0368563, Japan; imair@hirosaki-u.ac.jp
* Correspondence: a.momose@jusendo.or.jp

Received: 12 September 2019; Accepted: 11 November 2019; Published: 13 November 2019

Abstract: Background: We investigated ion channels at the skin, including peripheral nerve endings, which serve as output machines and molecular integrators of many pruritic inputs mainly received by multiple G protein-coupled receptors (GPCRs). **Methods:** Based on the level of chronic kidney disease–associated pruritus (CKD-aP), subjects were divided into two groups: non-CKD-aP (no or slight pruritus; n = 12) and CKD-aP (mild, moderate, or severe pruritus; n = 11). Skin samples were obtained from the forearm or elbow during operations on arteriovenous fistulas. We measured ion channels expressed at the skin, including peripheral nerve endings by RT-PCR: Nav1.8, Kv1.4, Cav2.2, Cav3.2, BK_{Ca}, Anoctamin1, TRPV1, TRPA1, and ASIC. **Results:** Expression of Cav3.2, BK_{Ca}, and anoctamin1 was significantly elevated in patients with CKD-aP. On the other hand, expression of TRPV1 was significantly reduced in these patients. We observed no significant difference in the levels of Cav2.2 or ASIC between subjects with and without CKD-aP. TRPA1, Nav1.8, and Kv1.4 were not expressed. **Conclusions:** It was concluded that this greater difference in the expression of ion channels in the skin tissue including, specially cutaneous peripheral nerve endings in CKD patients with CKD-aP may increase generator potential related to itching.

Keywords: uremic pruritus; ion channels; cell signaling; Cav3.2 calcium channel; RT-PCR; skin

1. Introduction

Itching can be caused by various stimuli, including mechanical, electrical, and chemical stimuli. Exogenous and endogenous chemical stimuli include amines, proteases, neuropeptides, inflammatory mediators, and certain drugs. However, in previous studies that compared immunostaining skin sections treated with various common pruritogens (histamine, acetylcholine (Ach), etc.), uremic substances, and other substances causing itching (e.g., β-endorphin and endothelin-1), no significant difference was observed between patients with and without CKD-aP, even though the immunostaining epidermis sections were stained regardless of CKD-aP [1].

Among uremic substances, for example, endothelin-1, which is classified of moderate molecular weight, and para-cresyl sulfate, a protein-bound uremic toxin, were reported as candidate substances that cause itching in patients with chronic kidney disease (CKD)-associated pruritus (CKD-aP) [2,3]. It is reported that uremic toxins stimulate the production of reactive oxygen species (ROS) and ROS act on ion channels which are associated with pruritus [4–7]. Although CKD patients undergo hemodialysis with a high-performance membrane or on-line hemodiafiltration, as well as long-term or frequent hemodialysis, to remove these uremic substances, approximately 40% of patients still suffer from CKD-aP [8].

These findings suggested that itching can be caused by receptors and other signals, instead of pruritogens. Therefore, we first examined the downstream ion channels because it is difficult to measure the complex and many downstream signals from ligands (pruritogens). Expressed ion channels in cutaneous peripheral nerve endings in healthy individuals are as follows: among the voltage-gated Na^+ channels (Nav), Nav1.7, Nav1.8, and Nav1.9; among the voltage-gated K^+ channels, Kv1.4, Kv3.4, and Kv7.2 (Kv); among the Ca^{2+}-activated K^+ channels (K_{Ca}), big conductance (BK_{Ca}); among the two-pore K^+ channels, TREK1 and TRAAK; among the voltage-gated Ca^+ channels (Cav), N-type (Cav2.2) and T-type (Cav3.2); among the Cl channels, calcium-activated chloride channel Anoctamin1 (TMEM16A); among the transient receptor potential (TRP) channels, TRP vanilloid 1 (TRPV1) and TRP ankyrin 1 (TRPA1); and acid-sensing ion channels (ASIC1) [9,10]. Among these channels, Nav1.8, Kv1.4, BK_{Ca}, Cav2.2, and Cav3.2 are expressed only in the cutaneous peripheral nerve endings, whereas TRPV1, TRPA1, Anoctamin1, BK_{Ca}, and ASIC are expressed not only in the peripheral nerve cells but also in keratinocytes at the skin.

Our goal was to test the hypothesis that many pruritogens including uremic toxins act on ion channels on the peripheral nerve endings directly or sensitize those via GPCRs and ROS indirectly, changing the output of multiple ion channels and increase generator potential and generate action potential related to CKD-aP, resulting in encoding the amplitude, frequency and quality of impulse of the peripheral nerve. To explore the peripheral neuronal mechanisms underlying itching, we compared the expression of several ion channels at the skin, including peripheral nerve endings between CKD patients with and without CKD-aP.

2. Materials and Methods

2.1. Subjects

This cohort-sectional study was approved by the Ethics Committee of Jusendo General Hospital. (Approval code: No.126). Each patient gave written informed consent. Between February 2016 and September 2018, we performed arteriovenous fistula surgery in 77 patients with CKD stage 5, either before the induction of hemodialysis (HD) or within 1 month after the induction of HD. Twenty-three patients (8 females and 15 males, 38–86 years old) and one control agreed to participate in the study. The control was a patient undergoing an operation for prostatic hypertrophy, who reported no pruritus. Patients with concomitant dermatitis, e.g., atopic dermatitis or psoriasis, were excluded. The degree of pruritus was determined according to Shiratori's Japanese classification of itching (Table 1). When the degree of pruritus was different between daytime and nighttime, a larger value of score was defined as the pruritus score. Based on the level of pruritus, subjects were divided into two groups: non-CKD-aP (no or slight pruritus; n = 12) and CKD-aP (mild, moderate, or severe pruritus; n = 11).

Table 1. Definitions of Shiratori's itch severity scores.

Score (Severity)	Daytime Symptoms	Nighttime Symptoms
4 (severe)	Intolerable itching, worsened instead of relieved by scratching. Cannot focus on work or study	Can hardly sleep because of itching. Scratching all the time, but itching intensifies with scratching
3 (moderate)	Scratching even in the presence of others. Irritation as a result of itching, continuous scratching	Wake up because of itching. Can fall asleep again after scratching, but continue to scratch unconsciously while sleeping
2 (mild)	Itch sensation is relieved by light, occasional scratching. Not too disturbing	Feel somewhat itchy, which is relieved by scratching. Do not wake up because of itch sensations
1 (slight)	Feel itchy sometimes, but tolerable without scratching	Feel slightly itchy when going to sleep, but do not need to scratch. Sleeping well
0 (no symptoms)	Hardly feel itchy or do not feel itchy at all	Hardly feel itchy or do not feel itchy at all

2.2. Study Designs

We compared age, gender, underlying disease, presence of hepatitis B or C, number of patients receiving treatment for itching, as well as levels of blood serum albumin, corrected Ca, inorganic phosphorus, intact parathyroid hormone (intact-PTH), blood serum hypersensitive C-reactive protein (hs-CRP), and blood ferritin in patients of the pruritus and non-pruritus groups.

Skin samples about 10×5 mm^2 were obtained from the forearm or elbow immediate after commencing operations on the arteriovenous fistulae.

2.3. Quantitative Real-Time Polymerase Chain Reaction (RT-PCR)

Expressed ion channels in cutaneous peripheral nerve endings in healthy individuals are as follows: among the voltage-gated Na$^+$ channels (Nav), Nav1.7, Nav1.8, and Nav1.9; among the voltage-gated K+ channels, Kv1.4, Kv3.4, and Kv7.2 (Kv); among the Ca^{2+}-activated K$^+$ channels (K$_{Ca}$), big conductance (BK$_{Ca}$); among the two-pore K+ channels, TREK1 and TRAAK; among the voltage-gated Ca$^+$ channels (Cav), N-type (Cav2.2) and T-type (Cav3.2); among the Cl channels, calcium-activated chloride channel Anoctamin1 (TMEM16A); among the transient receptor potential (TRP) channels, TRP vanilloid 1 (TRPV1) and TRP ankyrin 1 (TRPA1); and acid-sensing ion channels (ASIC1) [5,6]. Among the ion channels expressed in cutaneous peripheral nerve endings, we measured the levels of Nav1.8 (SCN10A), Kv1.4 (KCNA4), BK$_{Ca}$ (KCNMA1), Cav2.2 (CACNA 1B), Cav3.2 (CACNA 1H), Anoctamin1 (TREM16A), TRPV1, TRPA1, and ASIC by RT-PCR. Nav1.8, Kv1.4, Cav2.2, and Cav3.2 are expressed only in the cutaneous peripheral nerve endings, whereas TREM16A, TRPV1, TRPA1, ASIC1, and BK$_{Ca}$ are expressed not only in the peripheral nerve cells but also in keratinocytes at the skin.

Gene expression levels for ion channels were determined after reverse transcription of RNA samples by quantitative PCR by using an ABI PRISM 7000 Sequence Detector (Thermo Fisher Scientific, Waltham, MA, USA) as described previously [11]. Pre-made TaqMan® Gene Expression Assays for human were used (Table 2). Total RNA was isolated from the biopsied skin specimens with TRIzol (Thermo Fisher Scientific, Waltham, MA, USA). cDNA was synthesized from total RNA with reverse transcriptase reaction using SuperScript™ VILO™ Naster Mix (Thermo Fisher Scientific) following the manufacturer's protocol. cDNA was synthesized from 1 µg of total RNA. For standardization of quantitation, beta 2 microglobulin as amplified simultaneously. The expression level of each gene is presented as fold increase in the subjects showing itchy compared with control subject.

Table 2. Gene Assays ID.

Gene Name	Assay ID
ASIC1(acid sensing ion channel subunit 1)	Hs00952807_m1
Anoctamin 1	Hs00216121_m1
CACNA 1B (Cav2.2)	Hs04996252_m1
CACNA1H (Cav3.2)	Hs01103527_m1
KCNA4 (Kv1.4)	Hs00937357_s1
KCNMA1 (BK$_{Ca}$)	Hs01119504_m1
SCN10A (Nav1.8)	Hs01045151_m1
TRPA1	Hs00175798_m1
TRPV1	Hs00218912_m1
beta-2-microglobulin	Hs00187842_m1

Pre-made TaqMan® Gene Expression Assays for human were used (Thermo Fisher Scientific, Waltham, MA, USA).

2.4. Statistical Analysis

All values are expressed as means ± standard deviations (SD) for normally distributed data, medians (ranges) for non-normally distributed data, and numbers (percentages). No data points were excluded. All statistical analyses were performed using the unpaired *t*-test or m × n chi-square test for categorical outcomes. *p*-values < 0.05 were considered to be statistically significant.

3. Results

3.1. Baseline Characteristics

No differences were observed between the two groups in term of age, gender, underlying disease, duration of renal replacement therapy, presence of hepatitis B or C, number of patients receiving treatment for itching, or the levels of corrected Ca, inorganic phosphorus, blood serum albumin, blood serum hsCRP, and blood serum ferritin (Table 3).

Table 3. Patient characteristics.

Characteristic	Non-Pruritus (n = 12)	Pruritus (n = 11)	*p* Value
Degree of pruritus	none, slight	mild, moderate, severe	
Gender (F/M)	4/8	4/7	>0.05
Age (y.o.)	68 ± 10	68 ± 10	>0.05
Original disease (DM/CGN/PCK/unknown)	7/1/2/2	9/1/0/1	>0.05
HBV/HCV (n)	0/1	0/0	>0.05
Duration of HD (days)	23 (0–12779)	9 (0–5318)	>0.05
Albumin (d/dL)	3.2 ± 0.6	3.3 ± 0.4	>0.05
Corrected Ca (mg/dL)	8.8 ± 1.1	8.9 ± 0.6	>0.05
iP (mg/dl)	5.0 ± 1.8	5.7 ± 1.3	>0.05
i-PTH (pg/mL)	219 ± 126	233 ± 135	>0.05
hsCRP (mg/dL)	0.17 (0.02–1.44)	0.32 (0.04–8.00)	>0.05
Ferritin (ng/mL)	119 ± 84	130 ± 59	>0.05
Anti-pruritic therapy (nalfurafine, urea, predonisolone, crotamiton, diphenhydramine)	7 (58%)	3 (27%)	>0.05

Values are presented as means ± SD, median (range), or numbers (percentages). *p*-values were calculated using the unpaired t-test, Mann-Whitney U-test, or chi-square test. DM, diabetes mellitus; CGN, chronic glomeluronephritis; PCK, polycystic kidney; hsCRP, hypersensitivity C-reactive protein.

3.2. Analysis of Ion Channels at the Skin by RT-PCR

Expression of Cav3.2, BK_{Ca}, and Anoctamin1 was significantly higher in patients with CKD-aP. On the other hand, expression of TRPV1 was significantly decreased in those with CKD-aP. No significant difference in Cav2.2 and ASIC was observed between groups. TRPA1, Nav1.8, or Kv1.4 were not expressed (Table 4).

Table 4. Relative expression levels.

Gene Name		Non-Pruritus	Pruritus	*p*-Value
Cav3.2	CACNA 1H	0.948 (0.660–1.809) (n = 6)	2.490 (0.910–4.993) (n = 6)	0.039
Cav2.2	CACNA 1B	1.344 (0.038–19.186) (n = 5)	0.089 (0.066–0.977) (n = 3)	>0.05
Anoctamin1	TMEM 16A	1.094 (0.653–1.517) (n = 10)	1.528 (0.819–6.733) (n = 11)	0.009
ASIC1		0.796 (0.505–3.000) (n = 8)	2.962 (0.334–14.189) (n = 7)	>0.05
Kv1.4	KCNA4	No date	No date	
Na1.8	SCN10A	No date	No date	
TRPA1		No date	No date	
TRPV1		1.013 (0.804–1.223) (n = 3)	0.394 (0.256–0.463) (n = 3)	0.048
KCa1.1 (BK_{Ca})	KCNMA1	0.911 (0.526–1.685) (n = 7)	2.657 (0.664–4.042) (n = 7)	0.020

Values are expressed as median (range). *p*-values were calculated using the unpaired *t*-test. BK_{Ca}, large conductance in Ca^{2+}-activated K^+ channels.

4. Discussion

The primary receptors responsible for itch are G protein-coupled receptors (GPCRs) (approximately 800 types in human), which then transmit itch signals to trimeric proteins, effectors, second messengers, as well as targets [12]. These transmitted signals ultimately affect the expression or function (i.e., sensitization) of ion channels [13,14]. These ion channels depolarize receptor potentials, and action potentials occur when the total depolarized receptor potential exceeds the threshold of voltage-dependent Na+ channels. Consequently, peripheral nerve signals are encoded. These signals (impulses) are transmitted to the central nervous system, including the spinal cord and brain, resulting in itching and scratching. Therefore, ion channels seem to act as output machines and molecular integrators of many pruritic inputs, which are mainly received by multiple GPCRs.

The Cav3.2 T-type calcium channel, which is only expressed in peripheral nerves at the skin, is associated with depolarization (i.e., receptor potential), action potential generation, and itching [15]. Our study demonstrated that the expression of Cav3.2 T-type calcium channels was significantly higher in patients with CKD-aP compared to those without CKD-aP. Therefore, it was speculated that the threshold of itch in patients with CKD-aP decreased because the expression of Cav3.2 T-type calcium channels in the peripheral nerve endings increased. Many substances causing itching, such as histamine, up-regulate the Cav3.2 T-type Ca^{2+} channel via GPCR [16,17]. For example, a previous study reported that agonists of the ACh muscarinic receptor, which is a GPCR, increases T-currents in rats. This report suggested that the Cav3.2 T-type Ca^{2+} channel is associated with itching in patients with atopic disease who received ACh intradermally [18]. By contrast, another study reported that Cav3.2 T-type calcium channels are more sensitive to inhibition by metals, such as zinc, copper, and nickel [19]. Furthermore, the major natural and mammalian endogenous fatty acids, including γ-linolenic acid and arachidonic acid, as well as the fully polyunsaturated ω3-fatty acids that are enriched in fish oil are potent inhibitors of the Cav3.2 T-type calcium channels [20]. This inhibitory effect may allow some patients with CKD-aP to benefit from treatment with zinc, γ-linolenic acid (ω-3), and fully polyunsaturated ω3-fatty acids [21].

Ca3.2 T-channels regulate cellular excitability in the peripheral nerve endings of nociceptors, whereas Cav2.2 (N-type Ca^{2+} channels), which also is expressed in peripheral nerves, regulate the release of neurotransmitters such as glutamate and substance P in the central terminals of nociceptor neurons in the spinal dorsal horn [22]. No statistically significant difference was observed in expression of Cav2.2 calcium channels between patients with and without CKD-aP. These findings suggest that Cav2.2 calcium channels are mainly expressed on the central side of the peripheral nerve, not at ending side, and can be involved in the transmission pathway of the itching.

Nav1.8 contributes to action potential generation in dorsal root ganglion (DRG) neurons in mice. Also, voltage-gated potassium (Kv) channels shape action potentials by controlling the repolarization phase, and they also determine the membrane potential and duration of the inter-spike interval [23]. Based on these findings, we measured Nav1.8 and Kv1.4, which are also expressed only expressed in peripheral nerves at the skin [24], but neither Nav1.8 nor Kv1.4 were expressed in the cutaneous peripheral nerve ending in CKD patients. This suggested that Nav1.7 (PN1), Nav1.9 (PN5), or Kv7.1-Kv7.5 (KCNQ channels) may be more associated with CKD-aP.

TRPV1 are non-selective cation channels that act as biosensors for environmental and noxious stimuli, as well as changes in temperature and conditions inside the cell. In addition to capsaicin and resiniferatoxin (RTX), protons (pH < 5.7), heat (> 42 °C), and multiple other ligands (endogenous lipids and metabolic products of lipoxygenase) can directly activate TRPV1 [25,26] Furthermore, indirect activation of TRPV1 by pruritogens such as histamine appears to require an intracellular signal transduction mechanism that lies downstream of GPCRs (i.e., sensitization) [27]. TRPV1 expression was significantly lower in patients with CKD-aP. Because TRPV1 is expressed not only on sensory neurons, but also on keratinocytes and mast cells, reduced expression of TRPV1 in CKD patients with CKD-aP is not limited to the peripheral nerve ending. Given that cutaneous TRPV1 expression reflects its expression in cutaneous peripheral nerve endings, TRPV1 expression may be more associated with pain rather than itching, and indeed it may inhibit itching. Khomula et al. showed that the TRPV1 channels are down-regulated, and Cav3.2 T-type channels are up-regulated, under normalgesic types of peripheral diabetic neuropathy in streptozotocin-induced diabetes rats [28]. The pathophysiology of CKD-aP may be similar to that of peripheral diabetic neuropathy.

TRPA1, which is also expressed on cells other than peripheral nerve cells can be activated by various reactive compounds, including mustard oil, cinnamaldehyde, formalin, and hydrogen peroxide, as well as noxious cold temperature, reactive oxygen species (ROS), and inflammatory lipids (4-hydroxynonenol). Wilson et al. showed that TRPA1 is the downstream target of both mas-related GPCR (Mrgpr) A3 and Mrgprc11, which act as receptors for the pruritogens chloroquine and BAM8-22, respectively [29]. However, no TRPA1 expression was observed regardless of CKD-aP, suggesting that TRPA1 may be down-regulated by intracellular signals of itch such as H_2S [30]. Uremic toxins stimulate the production of ROS, such as H_2O_2, in mitochondria [4,5]. In addition, ROS sensitize Cav3.2 T-type calcium channels and Na^+ channels, as well as TRPA1 and TRPV, and also increase intracellular Ca^{2+} [6,7]. Thus, uremic toxins may be related to Cav3.2 T-type calcium channels through ROS as well as GPCRs.

In general, membrane depolarization increases the sensitivity of Anoctamin1 to an increase in intracellular Ca^{2+} [31]. Anoctamin1, which is also expressed not only on sensory neurons, but also on keratinocytes, further enhances the depolarization of receptor potentials by efflux of anion Cl^- from the cell [32]. Compared to patients without CKD-aP, Anoctamin1 expression increased in patients with CKD-aP. Given that cutaneous TRPV1 expression reflects its expression in cutaneous peripheral nerve endings, it was thought that sensitivity or expression of Anoctamin1 increased due to elevated intracellular Ca^{2+} via Cav3.2 T-type calcium channels.

There is evidence that members of the Cav3.2 T-type calcium channel can physically and functionally interact with the BK_{Ca} channels, which play a key role in controlling action potential repolarization [33]. BK_{Ca} expression, which is also expressed on cells other than peripheral nerve cells, was significantly increased in patients with CKD-aP due to the increase of intracellular Ca^{2+} through the Cav3.2 T-type calcium channel. If cutaneous BK_{Ca} expression reflects its expression in cutaneous peripheral nerve endings, this finding suggested that repolarization of action potentials, leading to itching, was activated; this might affect the shape or frequency of action potential impulses related to itching in cutaneous peripheral nerve ending. In fact, the frequency of itch impulses is less than that of pain impulses in peripheral c-fibers [34].

ASCI was higher in patients with CKD and H+ sensitivity than in healthy individuals, but the difference was not statistically significant, suggesting no direct impact of pH on CKD-aP.

Many times in the past a new treatment option has been reported to be effective, but very soon thereafter conflicting results appear. Most therapeutic trials have shown only limited success. We think that this is because pruritogens mainly act on ion channels indirectly through many GPCRs or ROS and do not act on ion channels directly such as on pain stimuli.

This cohort-sectional study had some limitations. First, the total number of samples were relatively small, which may restrict interpretation of our results. Due to the small number of subjects, it was divided into two groups (non-CKD-aP and CKD-aP) instead of five groups (no, slight, mild, moderate and severe pruritus group). However, this separating way may be less meaningful, because each pruritus has different molecular profile.

Second, we examined ion channels specifically expressed in peripheral nerve endings (e.g., Cav3.2) and those expressed in keratinocytes or other sites, as well as peripheral nerve ending (e.g., TRPV1). Presently, it is technically difficult to separate the peripheral nerves from skin cells and examine ion channels expressed only the peripheral nerve endings. This requires further research. We think that the combination of ion channel agonists and antagonists will lead to new drug discoveries in the future. In addition to expression studies, functional studies are also needed to investigate the physiological roles of these channels. There are many reports that increased membrane expression of the ion channel parallels functional up-regulation of the ion channel in neurons [35].

5. Conclusions

It was concluded that a greater difference was observed in expression of ion channels at the skin tissue including, specific, for cutaneous peripheral nerve endings in CKD patients with CKD-aP than in those without CKD-aP. This up-regulated expression of Cav3.2 T-type calcium channel of the peripheral nerve in patients with CKD-aP may increase the generator potential and induce action potentials related to itching.

Author Contributions: Conceptualization, A.M. and H.M.; methodology, A.M. and H.M.; formal analysis, A.M.; investigation, A.M., M.Y., S.C., H.M.; data curation, A.M., M.Y., and S.C.; writing—original draft preparation, A.M.; writing—review and editing, A.M., M.Y., S.C., and H.M., supervision, K.K., Y.S.

Funding: This research received no external fundings.

Acknowledgments: We thank Shun Susama, Takahiro Hirama and Takashi Kusakabe for their technical assistance, and Nobuhiko Takahashi, Hiroshi Toudoh, Masahiro Kanoh and Shunsuke Narita for discussions.

Conflicts of Interest: The authors declare no conflict of interest.

References

1. Momose, A.; Yabe, M.; Chiba, S.; Kumakawa, K.; Shiraiwa, Y.; Kusumi, T.; Mizukami, H. What are pruritogens of chronic kidney disease associated pruritus. *Acta Derm. Venereol.* **2017**, *97*, 1048.
2. Wang, C.P.; Lu, Y.C.; Tsai, I.T.; Tang, W.H.; Hsu, C.C.; Hung, W.C.; Yu, T.H.; Chen, S.C.; Chung, F.M.; Lee, Y.J.; et al. Increased levels of total p-cresylsulfate are associated with pruritus in patients with chronic kidney disease. *Dermatology* **2016**, *232*, 363–370. [CrossRef]
3. McQueen, D.S.; Noble, M.A.; Bond, S.M. Endothelin-1 activates ETA receptors to cause reflex scratching in BALB/c mice. *Br. J. Pharmacol.* **2007**, *151*, 278–284. [CrossRef] [PubMed]
4. Pieniazek, A.; Gwozdzinski, L.; Hikisz, P.; Gwozdzinski, K. Indoxyl sulfate generates free radicals, decreases antioxidant defense, and lead to damage to mononuclear blood cells. *Chem. Res. Toxicol.* **2018**, *31*, 869–875. [CrossRef] [PubMed]
5. Watanabe, H.; Miyamoto, Y.; Honda, D.; Tanaka, H.; Wu, Q.; Endo, M.; Noguchi, T.; Kadowaki, D.; Ishima, Y.; Kotani, S.; et al. p-Cresyl sulfate causes renal tubular cell damage by inducing oxidative stress by activation of NADPH oxidase. *Kidney Int.* **2013**, *83*, 582–592. [CrossRef] [PubMed]
6. Ogawa, N.; Kurokawa, T.; Mori, Y. Sensing of redox status by TRP channels. *Cell Calcium* **2016**, *60*, 115–122. [CrossRef] [PubMed]
7. Odorovic, S.M.; Jevtovic-Todorovic, V.; Meyenburg, A.; Mennerick, S.; Perez-Reyes, E.; Romano, C.; Olney, J.W.; Zorumski, C.F. Redox modulation of T-type calcium channels in rat peripheral nociceptors. *Neuron* **2001**, *31*, 75–85. [CrossRef]
8. Kimata, N.; Fuller, D.S.; Saitoh, A.; Akizawa, T.; Fukuhara, S.; Pisoni, R.L.; Robinson, B.M.; Akiba, T. Pruritus in hemodialysis patients: Results from the Japanese Dialysis Outcomes and Practive Patterns Study (JDOPPS). *Hemodial. Int.* **2014**, *18*, 657–667. [CrossRef] [PubMed]
9. Trantoulas, C.; McMahon, S.B. Opening paths to novel analgesics: The role of potassium channels in chronic pain. *Trends Neurosci.* **2014**, *37*, 146–158. [CrossRef]
10. Benarroch, E.E. Acid-sensing cation channels. *Neurology* **2014**, *82*, 628–635. [CrossRef]
11. Mizukami, H.; Mi, Y.; Wada, R.; Kono, M.; Yamashita, T.; Liu, Y.; Werth, N.; Sandhoff, R.; Proia, R.L. Systemic inflammation in glucocerebrosidase-deficient mice with minimal glucosylceramide storage. *J. Clin. Investig.* **2002**, *109*, 1215–1221. [CrossRef] [PubMed]
12. Geppetti, P.; Veldhuis, N.A.; Lieu, T.; Bunnett, N.W. G protein-coupled receptors: Dynamic machines for signaling pain and itch. *Neuron* **2015**, *88*, 635–649. [CrossRef] [PubMed]
13. Linley, J.E.; Rose, K.; Ooi, L.; Gamper, N. Understanding inflammatory pain. *Pflug. Arch.* **2010**, *459*, 657–669. [CrossRef] [PubMed]
14. Waxman, S.G.; Zamponi, G.W. Regulating excitability of peripheral afferents. *Nat. Neurosci.* **2014**, *17*, 153–163. [CrossRef]
15. Rose, K.E.; Lunardi, N.; Boscolo, A.; Dong, X.; Erisir, A.; Jevtovic-Todorovic, V.; Todorovic, S.M. Immunohistological demonstration of Cav3.2 T-type voltage-gated calcium channel expression in soma of dorsal ganglion neurons and peripheral axons of rat and mouse. *Neuroscience* **2013**, *250*, 263–274. [CrossRef]

16. Huc, S.; Monteil, A.; Bidaud, I.; Barbara, G.; Chemin, J.; Lory, P. Regulation of T-type calcium channels. *Biochim. Biophys. Acta* **2009**, *1793*, 947–952. [CrossRef]
17. Chemin, J.; Traboulsie, A.; Lory, P. Molecular pathways underlying the modulation of T-type calcium channels by neurotransmitters and hormones. *Cell Calcium* **2006**, *40*, 121–134. [CrossRef]
18. Heyer, G.; Vogelgsang, M.; Hornstein, O.P. Acethylcholine is an inducer of itching in patients with atopic eczema. *J. Dermatol.* **1997**, *24*, 621–625. [CrossRef]
19. Kang, H.W.; Vitko, I.; Lee, S.S.; Perez-Reyes, E.; Lee, J.H. Structural determinants of the high affinity extracellular zinc binding site on Cav3.2 T-type calcium channels. *J. Biol. Chem.* **2010**, *285*, 3271–3281. [CrossRef]
20. Mathie, A.; Sutton, G.L.; Clarke, C.E.; Veale, E.L. Zinc and copper. *Pharmacol. Ther.* **2006**, *111*, 567–583. [CrossRef]
21. Begum, R.; Belury, M.A.; Burgess, J.R.; Peck, L.W. Supplementation with n-3 and n-6 polyunsaturated fatty acids. *J. Ren. Nutr.* **2004**, *14*, 233–241. [CrossRef]
22. Zampoli, G.W.; Lewis, R.J.; Todorovic, S.M.; Arneric, S.P.; Snutch, T.P. Role of voltage-gated calcium channels in ascending pain pathways. *Brain Res. Rev.* **2009**, *60*, 84–89. [CrossRef] [PubMed]
23. Hille, B. (Ed.) The superfamily of voltage-gated channels. In *Ion Channels of Excitable Membranes*, 3rd ed.; Sinauer Press: Sunderland, MA, USA, 2001; pp. 61–92.
24. Renganathan, M.; Cummins, T.R.; Waxman, S.G. Contribution of Na(v)1.8 sodium channels to action potential electrogenesis in DRG neurons. *J. Neurophysiol.* **2001**, *86*, 629–640. [CrossRef] [PubMed]
25. Toth, B.I.; Szallasi, A.; Biro, T. Transient receptor potential channels and itch: How deep should we scratch? *Handb. Exp. Pharmacol.* **2015**, *226*, 89–133. [PubMed]
26. Taberner, F.J.; Fernandez-Ballester, G.; Fernandez-Carvajal, A.; Ferrer-Montiel, A. TRP channels interaction with lipids and its implications in disease. *Biochim. Biophys. Acta* **2015**, *1848*, 1818–1827. [CrossRef] [PubMed]
27. Veldhuis, N.A.; Poole, D.P.; Grace, M.; McIntyre, P.; Bunnett, N.W. The G protein-coupled receptor-transient receptor potential channel axis: Molecular insights for targeting disorders of sensation and inflammation. *Pharmacol. Rev.* **2015**, *67*, 36–73. [CrossRef] [PubMed]
28. Khomula, E.V.; Viatchenko-Karpinski, V.Y.; Borisyuk, A.L.; Duzhyy, D.E.; Belan, P.V.; Voitenko, N.V. Specific functioning of Cav3.2 T-type calcium and TRPV1 channels under different types of STZ-diabetic neuropathy. *Biochim. Biophys. Acta* **2013**, *1832*, 636–649. [CrossRef]
29. Wilson, S.R.; Gerhold, K.A.; Bifolck-Fisher, A.; Liu, Q.; Patel, K.N.; Dong, X.; Bautista, D.M. TRPA1 is required for histamine-independent, Mas-related g protein-coupled receptor-mediated itch. *Nat. Neurosci.* **2011**, *14*, 595–602. [CrossRef]
30. Hsu, C.C.; Kin, R.L.; Lee, L.Y.; Lin, Y.S. Hydrogen sulfade induces hypersensitivity of rat capsaicin-sensitive lung vagal neurons. *Am. J. Physiol. Regul. Integr Comp. Physiol.* **2013**, *305*, 769–779. [CrossRef]
31. Benarroch, E.E. Anoctamins (TMEM16 proteins). *Neurology* **2017**, *89*, 722–729. [CrossRef]
32. Sun, X.; Gu, X.Q.; Haddad, G.G. Calcium influx via L- and N-type calcium channels activates a transient large-conductance Ca^{2+}-activated K^+ current in mouse neocortical pyramidal neurons. *J. Neurosci.* **2003**, *23*, 3639–3648. [CrossRef] [PubMed]
33. Pedemonte, N.; Galietta, L.J.V. Structure and function of TMEM16 proteins (anoctamins). *Physiol. Rev.* **2014**, *94*, 419–459. [CrossRef] [PubMed]
34. Hees, J.; Gybels, J. C nociceptor activity in human nerve during painful and non painful skin stimulation. *J. Neurosurg. Psychiatry* **1981**, *44*, 600–607. [CrossRef] [PubMed]
35. Liu, Q.Y.; Chen, W.; Cui, S.; Liao, F.F.; Yi, M.; Liu, F.Y.; Wan, Y. Upregulation of Cav3.2 T-type calcium channels in adjacent intact L4 dorsal root ganglion neurons in neuropathic pain rats with L5 spinal nerve ligation. *Neurosci. Res.* **2019**, *142*, 30–37. [CrossRef]

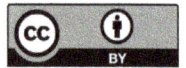

© 2019 by the authors. Licensee MDPI, Basel, Switzerland. This article is an open access article distributed under the terms and conditions of the Creative Commons Attribution (CC BY) license (http://creativecommons.org/licenses/by/4.0/).

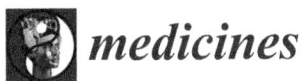

Perspective

Itch in Chronic Wounds: Pathophysiology, Impact, and Management

Michela Iannone [1,*], Agata Janowska [1], Valentina Dini [1], Giulia Tonini [1], Teresa Oranges [1,2] and Marco Romanelli [1]

[1] Department of Dermatology, University of Pisa, 56126 Pisa, Italy; agatina82@gmail.com (A.J.); valentinadini74@gmail.com (V.D.); giuliatonini19@gmail.com (G.T.); teresa.oranges@gmail.com (T.O.); romanellimarco60@gmail.com (M.R.)
[2] Department of Health Sciences, Anna Meyer Children's University Hospital, University of Florence, 50139 Florence, Italy
* Correspondence: drmichelaiannone@gmail.com; Tel.: +39-050-992-436; Fax: +39-050-992-556

Received: 30 June 2019; Accepted: 13 November 2019; Published: 15 November 2019

Abstract: Background: The aims of this review are to analyze the current literature regarding the characteristics and pathophysiological mechanisms of itch in chronic wounds, to assess the impact on quality of life and delayed-healing, to focus on the best strategies of prevention and treatment, to highlight the importance of on-going research in order to fully understand the pathophysiology, and to improve the management of target therapies. **Methods:** A systematic literature review was performed using MEDLINE, PubMed, Embase, Scopus, ScienceDirect, and the Cochrane Library. We included a total of 11 articles written in English with relevant information on the pathophysiology of itch in chronic wounds and on management strategies. **Results:** Itch in chronic wounds was found to be correlated with xerosis, larger wound areas, necrotic tissue and amount of exudate, peripheral tissue edema, sclerosis, granulation tissue, contact dermatitis, and bacterial burden, as well as with lower quality of life. **Conclusions:** Although there are several aspecific pharmacological and non-pharmacological approaches, there appears to be no validated prevention or management strategy for itch in chronic wounds. Further studies are needed to clarify the association and pathophysiology of itch in chronic wounds, to evaluate the safety and efficacy of topical treatments on perilesional skin to reduce itch, to characterize multidimensional sensations of itch in chronic wounds, to identify specific cytokine and chemokine expressions that are correlated to a tailored-based approach, and to develop practical guidelines.

Keywords: chronic pruritus; itch; pruritus; wounds; itch in wounds; itch management

1. Introduction

Itch is a chief symptom in many dermatological diseases, which significantly impacts patients' quality of life (QoL) [1]. Few studies, however, have analyzed the clinical itch characteristics and pathophysiological mechanisms of itch in chronic wounds [2–12]. Thus, the aim of this review is to analyze the current literature on the characteristics and pathophysiological mechanisms of itch in chronic wounds, to assess the impact on QoL and delayed wound healing, and to focus on prevention and treatment strategies for pruritus associated with chronic wounds.

2. Methods

Literature Search

A systematic literature search was performed to identify major findings on itch in chronic wounds in adults. We used the following databases: MEDLINE, PubMed, Embase, Scopus, ScienceDirect, and the Cochrane Library. The search included all studies published between January 2000 and June 2019. Keywords used were: itch in wounds, itch in leg ulcers, itch, chronic venous disease, wound pruritus, chronic wound itch, and itch management. We included only articles in English, with relevant information on the pathophysiology of wound-related itch and on management strategies. We excluded case reports, pediatric articles, and articles on acute wounds such as post-burn wounds.

We included a total of 11 articles.

The PRISMA 2019 flow diagram shown in Figure 1 explains the search methodology used in the study.

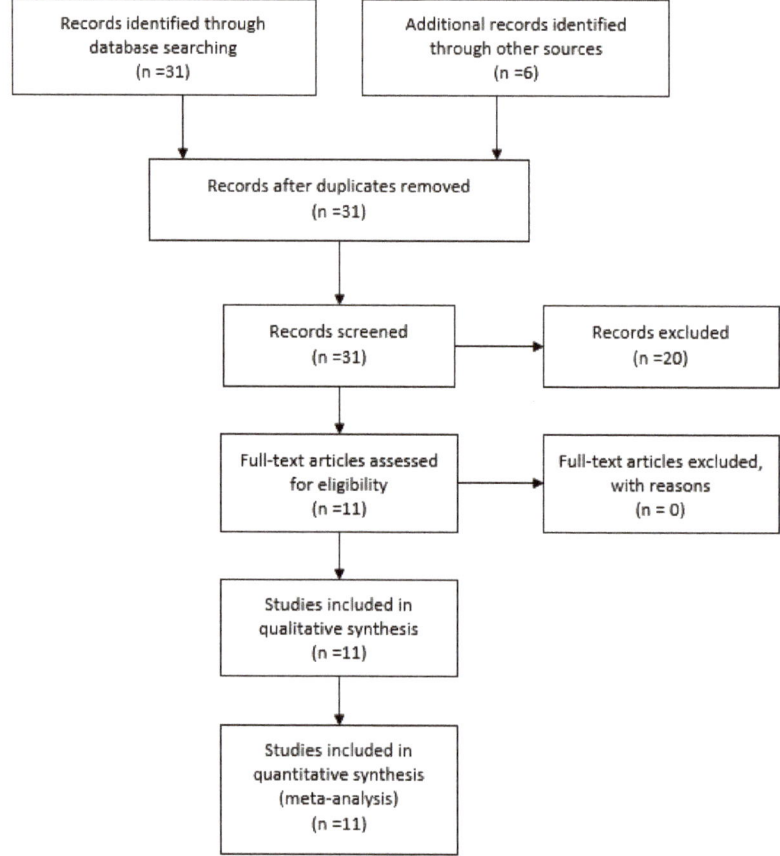

Figure 1. PRISMA flow diagram showing the literature search on itch in wounds.

3. Results

3.1. Characteristics and Pathophysiological Mechanisms of Itch

We selected nine articles focused on the characteristics and pathophysiological mechanisms of itch. Table 1 summarizes the main key data—authors, year of publication, country, type of article, purpose of the study, and findings [4–12].

Table 1. Key data from literature review.

Authors	Year	Country	Type of Article	Purpose of Study	Findings
Hareendran A. et al. [2]	2005	United Kingdom	Qualitative and quantitative methods were used to explore health related quality of life (HRQoL) issues in 38 patients	Identify HRQoL issues in patients with venous leg ulcers	Itching was reported in 69.4% of patients but no influence on sleep and functional limitations were found
Hareendran A. et al. [3]	2007	United Kingdom	In-depth interviews with focus group of 36 patients	To develop and validate a disease-specific quality of life (QoL) measure, based on the conceptual model of the Skin Disease impact on quality of life Index (SKINDEX-29) for patients with chronic venous leg ulcers	Itch was ranked 4th among ten symptoms causing distress in chronic venous ulcers
Paul J.C. et al. [4]	2011	Michigan (USA)	Cross sectional study on 161 patients	Investigate itch related to chronic venous disease, pain, and QoL.	Positive correlation between intensity of itch and severity of venous disease with lower QoL
Paul J. [5]	2013	Michigan (USA)	Cross sectional study on 199 patients with chronic wounds of different etiologies	Comparing pain and itch in chronic wounds	Wound-related itch was significantly associated with age, xerosis, employment status, and with venous wounds. Itch was rated higher on the perilesional skin, while pain was rated higher on the wound bed.
Paul J. [6]	2013	Michigan (USA)	Observational study on 200 patients with chronic wounds of different etiologies	Explore characteristics of wound-related itch	Itch characterizes more severe wounds with larger size, more tissue edema, and granulation issue and was also associated with moderate exudate amount or necrotic tissue
Upton D. et al. [7]	2013	United Kingdom	Literature review	Overview of the physiological mechanisms of itch and comorbidities in acute and chronic wounds	The itch causes a range of physical and psychological problems, reducing QoL and delaying healing. There are no specific guidelines on itch management in chronic wounds and further studies are needed.
Upton D. et al. [8]	2013	Australia	Literature review	Overview on psychological itch treatment in wounds	Unconventional treatments such as habit reversal training, relaxation, massage, and itch coping programs showed a potential role in reducing itch in association with standard treatments, but current literature evidence is limited.
D'Erme A.M. et al. [9]	2016	Italy	Literature review	Overview on contact allergy and polysensitization in patients with chronic wounds	Advanced dressings can cause allergic contact dermatitis. The most frequent was hydrogel, followed by hydrocolloid and by silver wound dressings. Primary prevention is required, avoiding sensitizers and irritant products, along with secondary prevention using patch tests in all patients with non-healing wounds.

Table 1. *Cont.*

Authors	Year	Country	Type of Article	Purpose of Study	Findings
Paul J. [10]	2018	Michigan (USA)	Structured interviews of 199 patients with chronic wounds	Identify descriptors for wound-related itch	15 descriptors identified (annoying, bothersome, just want itching to go away, unpleasant, stubborn, disturbing sleep, insistent, disgusting, severe, awful, prickly, warm, worrisome, unbearable, uncontrollable)
Parnell L.K.S. et al. [11]	2018	Texas (USA)	Literature review	Overview on itch research focusing on itch in wound care	Importance of multidimensional questionnaires to characterize itch. The authors described sensory, affective dimensions of itch, the itch trigger, and itch receptors and pathways. They highlighted both conventional and unconventional pharmacological therapies.
Lerner E. [12]	2018	South Carolina (USA)	Literature review	Overview of current understanding on the physiology of itch in wounds	Proposal for unconventional therapeutic approaches based on physiology

3.2. Impact on QoL

We selected four articles regarding the impact on QoL. The key data are summarized in Table 1 [2–4,7].

3.3. Prevention of Itch in Chronic Wounds

We found no articles on how to prevent itch in chronic wounds, so we decided to correlate data on the pathophysiological mechanisms of itch with current wound care management strategies.

4. Discussion

Cutaneous chronic wounds are classified as vascular (arterial, venous, mixed arterial-venous), diabetic foot ulcers, pressure ulcers, and atypical wounds (such as inflammatory, neoplastic, vasculitis, and exogenous). Wound itch is a frequent problem in clinical practice, but is poorly described in the literature. There are currently no exact data on the incidence and/or prevalence of itch in cutaneous wounds. The only data available report the characteristics of wounds and their relationship with itch. Our results from the systematic review show a linear correlation between wound area and itch through the release of itch triggers such as histamine and growth factors on the wound bed [6].

Remaining on wound characteristics analysis, the amount of necrotic wound bed tissue is another important finding; dead tissue blocks healing and leads to scratching, with further damage and enlargement of wounds [6].

A high amount of exudate is another wound characteristic that causes maceration and is an itch trigger factor. The collection of fluids in tissue can also causes mechanical stress that may exacerbate itch and promote mast cell invasion into nerve fibers, which can trigger or aggravate itch [6].

The induration in the periwound area, i.e., sclerosis, is another potential cause of wound itch; tissue damage activates inflammatory processes with mast cell degranulation promoting the release of pruritogen mediators [7].

The final findings of our review are about the granulation tissue. This tissue occurs in the proliferative phase of the wound healing process and contains fibroblasts and different types of inflammatory cells and may also release neoangiogenesis factors, connective proteins, nerve growth factors, and pruritogen mediators, which partially explain the phrase "it's itching, it must be healing", commonly used by healthcare providers [6]. However in some conditions, such as in infected wounds, granulation tissue can be hypertrophic and friable, and can cause excessive itch. Infected wounds may also itch because bacterial biofilm can interact through proadrenomedullin N-terminal 20 peptide (PAMP) with Toll-like 2 receptors (TLR-2, and activate protein cascades with the release of itch mediators [13].

Regarding management, the tissue debridement, inflammation/infection, moisture imbalance, epithelial edge advancement (TIME) principles of wound bed preparation are particularly effective in the management of these pathophysiologic factors in order to reduce the itch sensation [14].

By correlating the level of itch with wound management, our literature review has shown that, in selected patients, moderate compression bandaging can be used to manage itch by increasing the venous tone and normalizing circulation by removing edema [15].

Another important itch management strategy is the proper care of perilesional skin by two steps: proper selection of the wound dressings in line with the level of exudate and the size of the wound and the utilization of barrier products (principally zinc oxide paste, silicone-based ointments, polymer barrier preparations) and moisturizers [16].

If causative treatment fails, a stepwise therapeutic approach based on the European S2k Guideline on Chronic Pruritus is recommended. Step 1 consists of moisturizers and emollients containing urea (5%–10%), glycerol (20%), camphor (2%), menthol (1%), zinc (10%), pramoxine (1%), and polidocanol, and in systemic therapies with anti-h1 non-sedating antihistamines. Step 2 consists of topical anti-inflammatories (steroids and calcineurin inhibitors), gabapentinoids, and mu-opioid receptor antagonists. Step 3 consists of adding selected antidepressants (paroxetine, mirtazapine, doxepin, amitriptyline) or neurokinin receptor 1 antagonists [17].

5. Conclusions

Itch in wounds is a very frequent symptom and should never be underestimated. A better characterization of itch in chronic wounds and the identification of best strategies of prevention and treatment would improve the daily functions, the psychological state, and the social interactions of patients affected by chronic wounds.

The pathophysiology is particularly complex and multifactorial, and it is not fully understood. Numerous factors influence itch such as wound area, necrotic tissue amount, exudate amount, peripheral tissue edema, sclerosis, granulation tissue, bacterial biofilm, chronic venous insufficiency (CVI), perilesional skin characteristics, neuropathic changes, and dressing sensitization, as well as by psychological and emotional components. An itch-scratch cycle can lead to secondary infections, changes in pigmentation, thickening of the skin, and delayed healing.

The subjective and multidimensional nature of itch makes it a real challenge for clinicians. Various assessment tools have been used to evaluate itch. A critical point of further research is a consensus on the development of structured questionnaires to evaluate and measure the sensory and affective dimensions of itch in chronic wounds.

Currently, there are no standards for preventing and managing itch in chronic wounds. The TIME principles of wound bed preparation, the topical management of perilesional skin, and a stepwise therapeutic approach based on European S2k Guideline on chronic itch (if causative treatment has failed) seem to be the best management strategies to date.

Our study presents some methodological limitations. First, the literature data on the physiopathology and management of itch in chronic wounds was particularly poor. Second, itch has very complex underlying mechanisms of a subjective and multidimensional nature, which made our investigation complicated. Third, our literature review was limited to data available on online databases.

Further studies are needed to clarify the association and pathophysiology of itch in chronic wounds, and to evaluate the safety and efficacy of topical treatments on perilesional skin and of moderate compression to reduce itch. Further research on correlations among severity of itch and cytokines, chemokines, and inflammatory marker levels in exudates, perilesional, and lesional skin in different healing phases would help in developing targeted therapies for itch in chronic wounds.

Such studies should adopt a tailored-based approach and draw up practical guidelines.

The take-home messages of this review are summarized in Table 2.

Table 2. Take-home messages.

Take-Home Messages
✓ Itch in wounds is a very frequent symptom and should never be underestimated. The underlying mechanisms are very complex, including those of a subjective and multidimensional nature, which make investigations a real challenge for clinicians.
✓ The application of the tissue debridement, inflammation/infection, moisture imbalance, epithelial edge advancement (TIME) principles of wound bed preparation, the topical management of perilesional skin, and a stepwise therapeutic approach based on European S2k Guideline on chronic itch (if causative treatment fails) seem to be the best management strategies to date.
✓ Further studies are needed to better characterize and develop targeted therapies for itch in chronic wounds, adopting a tailored-based approach and drawing up practical guidelines.

Author Contributions: M.I. wrote the paper; T.O., M.R. and V.D. proofread the manuscript; A.J. and G.T. helped select and review the articles.

Funding: This research received no external funding.

Conflicts of Interest: The authors declare no conflict of interest.

References

1. Brenaut, E.; Garlantezec, R.; Talour, K.; Misery, L. Itch Characteristics in Five Dermatoses: Non-atopic Eczema, Atopic Dermatitis, Urticaria, Psoriasis and Scabies. *Acta Derm. Venereol.* **2013**, *93*, 573–574. [CrossRef] [PubMed]
2. Hareendran, A.; Bradbury, A.; Budd, J.; Geroulakos, G.; Hobbs, R.; Kenkre, J.; Symonds, T. Measuring the impact of venous leg ulcers on quality of life. *J. Wound Care* **2005**, *14*, 53–57. [CrossRef] [PubMed]
3. Hareendran, A.; Doll, H.; Wild, D.J.; Moffatt, C.J.; Musgrove, E.; Wheatley, C.; Franks, P.J. The venous leg ulcer quality of life (VLU-QoL) questionnaire: Development and psychometric validation. *Wound Repair Regen.* **2007**, *15*, 465–473. [CrossRef] [PubMed]
4. Paul, J.C.; Pieper, B.; Templin, T.N. Itch: Association with chronic venous disease, pain, and quality of life. *J. Wound Ostomy Continence Nurs.* **2011**, *38*, 46–54. [CrossRef] [PubMed]
5. Paul, J. A cross-sectional study of chronic wound-related pain and itching. *Ostomy Wound Manage* **2013**, *59*, 28–34. [PubMed]
6. Paul, J. Characteristics of chronic wounds that itch. *Adv. Skin Wound Care* **2013**, *26*, 320–332. [CrossRef] [PubMed]
7. Upton, D.; Richardson, C.; Andrews, A.; Rippon, M. Wound pruritus: Prevalence, aetiology and treatment. *J. Wound Care* **2013**, *22*, 501–508. [CrossRef] [PubMed]
8. Upton, D.; Penn, F.; Richardson, C.; Rippon, M. Psychological management of wound pruritus. *J. Wound Care* **2014**, *23*, 291–299. [CrossRef] [PubMed]
9. D'Erme, A.M.; Iannone, M.; Dini, V.; Romanelli, M. Contact dermatitis in patients with chronic leg ulcers a common and neglected problem: A review 2000–2015. *J. Wound Care* **2016**, *25*, S23–S29. [CrossRef] [PubMed]
10. Paul, J. Descriptors for Itch Related to Chronic Wounds. *Wounds* **2018**, *30*, 4–9. [PubMed]
11. Parnell, L.K.S. Itching for Knowledge About Wound and Scar Pruritus. *Wounds* **2018**, *30*, 17–36. [PubMed]
12. Lerner, E. Why Do Wounds Itch? *Wounds* **2018**, *30*, 1–3. [PubMed]
13. Gardner, S.E.; Frantz, R.A. Wound bioburden and infection. In *Wound Care Essentials: Practice Principles*, 3rd ed.; Baranoski, S., Ayello, E.A., Eds.; Lippincott Williams & Wilkins: Philadelphia, PA, USA, 2012; Volume 1, pp. 126–174.
14. Schultz, G.S.; Sibbald, R.G.; Falanga, V.; Ayello, E.A.; Dowsett, C.; Harding, K.; Romanelli, M.; Stacey, M.C.; Teot, L.; Vanscheidt, W. Wound bed preparation: A systematic approach to wound management. *Wound Repair Regen.* **2003**, *11*, S1–S28. [CrossRef] [PubMed]
15. Duque, M.I.; Yosipovitch, G.; Chan, Y.H.; Smith, R.; Levy, P. Itch, pain, and burning sensation are common symptoms in mild to moderate chronic venous insufficiency with an impact on quality of life. *J. Am. Acad. Dermatol.* **2005**, *53*, 504–508. [CrossRef] [PubMed]
16. Gray, M.; Weir, D. Prevention and treatment of moisture-associated skin damage (maceration) in the periwound skin. *J. Wound Ostomy Continence Nurs.* **2007**, *34*, 153–157. [CrossRef] [PubMed]
17. Weisshaar, E.; Szepietowski, J.C.; Dalgard, F.J.; Garcovich, S.; Gieler, U.; Giménez-Arnau, A.M.; Lambert, J.; Leslie, T.; Mettang, T.; Misery, L.; et al. European S2k Guideline on Chronic Pruritus. *Acta Derm. Venereol.* **2019**, *99*, 469–506. [CrossRef] [PubMed]

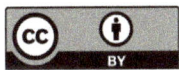

© 2019 by the authors. Licensee MDPI, Basel, Switzerland. This article is an open access article distributed under the terms and conditions of the Creative Commons Attribution (CC BY) license (http://creativecommons.org/licenses/by/4.0/).

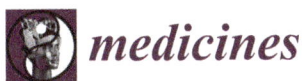

Review

Breaking the Itch–Scratch Cycle: Topical Options for the Management of Chronic Cutaneous Itch in Atopic Dermatitis

Ian P. Harrison and Fabrizio Spada *

Department of Research and Development, Ego Pharmaceuticals Pty Ltd., 21-31 Malcolm Road, Braeside VIC 3195, Australia
* Correspondence: fabrizio.spada@egopharm.com; Tel.: +61-03-9586-8874

Received: 20 June 2019; Accepted: 16 July 2019; Published: 18 July 2019

Abstract: Chronic itch is an unpleasant sensation that triggers a desire to scratch that lasts for six weeks or more. It is a major diagnostic symptom of myriad diseases, including atopic dermatitis for which it is the most prominent feature. Chronic itch can be hugely debilitating for the sufferer, damaging in terms of both the monetary cost of treatment and its socioeconomic effects, and few treatment options exist that can adequately control it. Corticosteroids remain the first line treatment strategy for atopic dermatitis, but due to the risks associated with long-term use of corticosteroids, and the drawbacks of other topical options such as topical calcineurin inhibitors and capsaicin, topical options for itch management that are efficacious and can be used indefinitely are needed. In this review, we detail the pathophysiology of chronic pruritus, its key features, and the disease most commonly associated with it. We also assess the role of the skin and its components in maintaining a healthy barrier function, thus reducing dryness and the itch sensation. Lastly, we briefly detail examples of topical options for the management of chronic pruritus that can be used indefinitely, overcoming the risk associated with long-term use of corticosteroids.

Keywords: chronic pruritus; skin; atopic dermatitis; ceramide; pine tar

1. Introduction: the Pathophysiology of Pruritus

Itch, formally "pruritus" from the Latin "prurit" ("to itch"), has been defined as "an unpleasant cutaneous sensation which provokes the desire to scratch" [1]. It is a common response to many stimuli, and a feature of many diseases, from systemic conditions such as renal insufficiency [2] to skin diseases such as atopic dermatitis (AD), of which itch is *the* major symptom [3,4]. Unlike acute itch, which is transient and usually overcome quickly by scratching the affected area, chronic itch is persistent and debilitating, to the point that the act of scratching can actually aggravate the problem even while providing relief [5]. While there are many treatment options available for chronic cutaneous pruritus, most are unsatisfactory due to the complex nature of the itch response and the subjective nature of the problem itself. The mere thought of itching can confound treatment outcomes: mentioning itch to a person will usually elicit an itch response in them that could damage the skin further, even if the treatment is successfully dealing with the underlying condition. Indeed, the effect of psychology can make it extremely difficult to assess the efficacy of antipruritic agents: it has been noted that the placebo effect can be as high as 50% in pruritus patients [6]. Successful management strategies ideally should incorporate into the chosen treatment regimen the daily use of easily-accessible, efficacious topical preparations designed primarily to tackle the itch. The benefits of these products could conceivably be twofold: physically alleviating the itch stimulus while helping to overcome the psychological need to scratch by allowing for the *ad libitum* application of the product. This review aims to provide a brief overview of itch, its impact in atopic dermatitis, and detail the components of the stratum corneum

1.1. Classifying Itch

Itch can be broadly classified into four distinct clinical categories: neurogenic, neuropathic, psychogenic and pruritoceptive [7]. Experiencing itch from one of these categories does not preclude the sufferer from experiencing an additional one or more other categories of itch concurrently. Neurogenic itch stems from disorders affecting organ systems, such as renal failure [8] and liver disease [9], while neuropathic itch can be a result of lesions on or pathological changes to the afferent pathway signaling to the central nervous system [10]. Psychogenic itch refers to itch associated with psychological maladies that do not have an underlying physiological etiology, such as delusional parasitosis [10]. The most common category of itch, and the category of note to this review, is pruritoceptive or cutaneous itch, an itch caused by inflammation of the skin [11]. This inflammation can be localized and transient as a result of, say, an insect bite, or it can be chronic and widespread as a result of disease. The fact that cutaneous pruritus is so common can be attributed to the nature of the skin itself: as the body's barrier to the external environment, the skin is subject to the effects of both endogenous mediators of itch (inflammation for example) and exogenous allergens, irritants and mechanical disruption.

1.2. Neural Mechanisms of Itch

The exact mechanisms of itch are poorly understood, such is its complexity. Numerous theories exist to try to explain pruriceptive sensation, notably the specificity and the pattern theories. The specificity theory posits that there are specific nerve fibers and neurons that transmit the itch response to the central nervous system (CNS), whereas the pattern theory suggests that itch is encoded across numerous sensory receptors and neurons, and that the pattern of this neuronal activity is what determines the sensation that is experienced [12,13]. Currently, the literature seems to favor the specificity theory [14].

The perception of itch starts when an itch-causing substance, or pruritogen, enters through the stratum corneum and binds to its receptors on sensory afferent nerves, or C-fibers, which transmit the resulting signal to the CNS where the brain interprets it as an itch and initiates a scratch response. Endogenous pruritogens can also be produced by both keratinocytes and immune cells such as mast cells, which produce histamine, a key mediator of itch (Figure 1). The distribution, thickness and density of intraepidermal nerve fibers is much higher in AD skin, which may exacerbate the itch response [15].

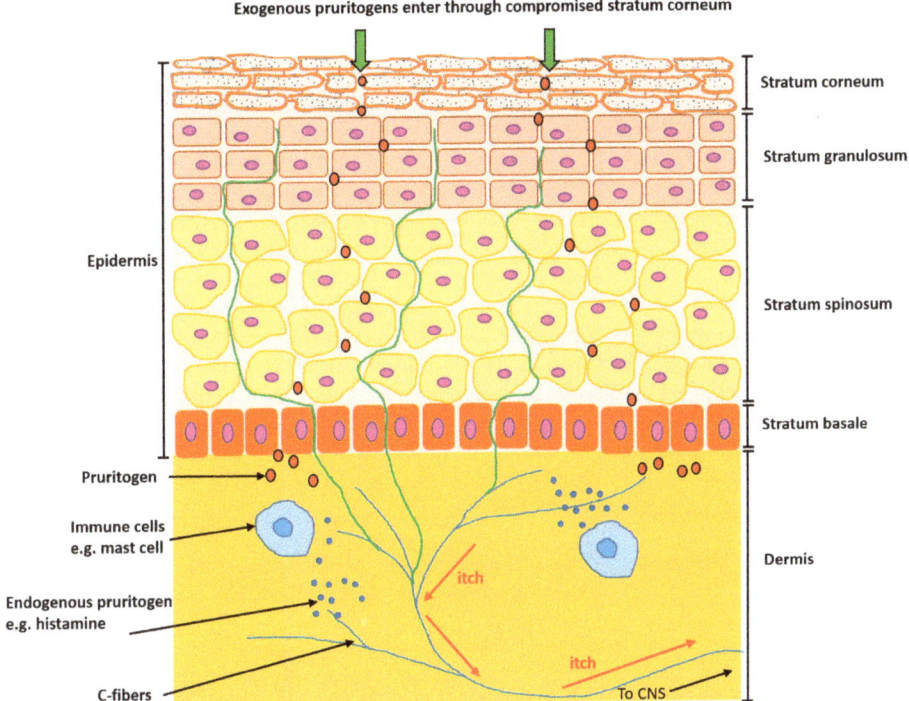

Figure 1. The itch pathway. Exogenous itch-causing substances, pruritogens, enter through the compromised stratum corneum and journey through the layers of the skin until they bind to their receptors on sensory afferent nerves, or C-fibers (in blue), triggering a signal which travels up the central nervous system (CNS) to the brain, where it is recognized as an itch. In addition, endogenous pruritogens such as histamine can be produced by cells of the body, such as mast cells. Nerve distribution and density is increased within the epidermis in AD skin (in green).

1.3. Endogenous Mediators of Pruritus

In addition to exogenous mediators of pruritus, numerous endogenous biological mediators exist that can elicit a pruritoceptive response in the skin. First and foremost is histamine, the most commonly used experimental pruritogen. Histamine is primarily produced by dermal mast cells in response to allergic stimuli, hence the first-line use of antihistamines as treatments for allergies. Histamine binds four known receptors, H1 to H4, with H1 being the primary receptor subtype responsible for itch. These receptors are located on sensory neurons, which transmit the signal created by the activated receptors to the brain to be recognized as itch. Crucially for AD, however, is that it is non-histaminergic itch pathways that are thought to predominate in the disease. A 2017 study of patients with AD found that itch sensation to cowhage, a tropical legume native to Asia and Africa and a potent pruritogen, was significantly greater both intra- and extralesionally than control compared with itch responses to histamine, which were not significantly different in AD skin versus control skin [16]. The monoamine neurotransmitter serotonin and the vasodilator bradykinin, while both relatively non-pruritogenic in normal skin, elicit strong pruritic responses in AD skin that are also histamine-independent [17]. Endogenous serine proteases such as tryptase are known to elicit an itch response, and are also upregulated in AD skin [18,19]. Interleukin-31 (Il-31), a Th2 cytokine of the IL-6 family of cytokines, is another prominent endogenous mediator of pruritus, especially in AD skin. Elevated levels of IL-31 have been observed in AD skin [20], and IL-31 receptor A expression is also most abundant in the dorsal root ganglia, the primary site of cutaneous sensory neurons [20]. A 2018 meta-analysis of studies looking at Il-31 in AD found that serum levels of IL-31 are proportional to the severity of AD, with the greatest levels of serum IL-31 in patients with severe AD [21].

2. The Stratum Corneum, Atopic Dermatitis and Pruritus

The stratum corneum, the outermost layer of the skin, forms the protective barrier between the inner body and the outside world [22]. Its barrier functions are numerous, from the prevention of trans-epidermal water loss from the epidermis to the external environment, to protection from external pathogens. It is composed of approximately 15–25 layers of dead, flattened keratinocytes (corneocytes) embedded in a lipid bilayer [23], which gives rise to the "brick and mortar" model most commonly used to describe it [24]. The lipid bilayer consists of approximately 50% ceramides, 25% cholesterol and 10–15% free fatty acids, with small amounts of glucosylceramides and phospholipids [24]. Instead of the plasma membrane that encases living cells, corneocytes are surrounded by an insoluble cornified cell envelope composed of a monolayer of ceramides, and are held together in the lipid bilayer by corneodesmosomes, modified desmosomes from the uppermost layer of the stratum granulosum [25] (Figure 2).

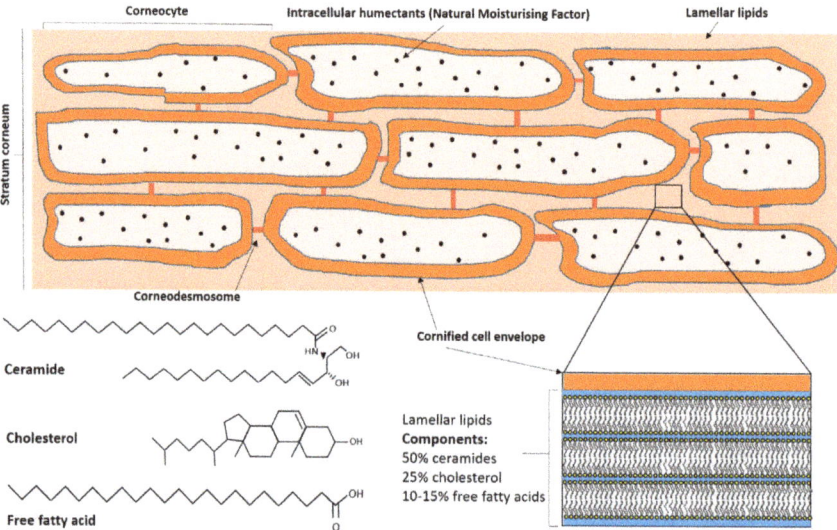

Figure 2. Schematic representation of the stratum corneum, with a view of the composition of the lamellar lipid layer. The typical chemical compositions of the major skin barrier lipids (ceramides, cholesterol and free fatty acids) are shown at bottom left.

AD, the most common chronic inflammatory skin disease, affects up to 3% of adults and up to 20% of children worldwide [26], with its incidence increasing in developing countries [27]. While the pathophysiology of AD is complex and not entirely understood, it is universally acknowledged that an essential symptom and diagnostic feature of the disease is the intense chronic itch [28]. The itch, combined with the scratching it necessitates, exacerbates the morbidity of the disease and can lead to physical damage: the act of scratching compromises the integrity of the skin, damaging that crucial barrier to the outside world. This damaged barrier essentially becomes an open border, allowing for passage through it from either side: the skin of AD sufferers is extremely dry, owing to the loss of moisture [29], but it also tends to be more susceptible to infection, as external pathogens take advantage of the damaged barrier and compromised immune function [30]. In addition, the dysfunctional barrier seen in AD also results in enhanced antigen penetration, leading to exacerbated allergic reactions. Moisture loss and pathogen infiltration exacerbates dryness and can lead to inflammation, perpetuating the need to scratch, which itself further damages the skin barrier, exacerbates dryness and increases pro-inflammatory mediator release. This sequence of events is commonly referred to as the "itch–scratch cycle" [31,32]. In addition to the physical damage, the itch–scratch cycle can also lead to debilitating psychological sequelae. AD has been associated with depression, anxiety and suicidal ideation, with the severity of these psychiatric diseases proportional to the severity of AD [33]. The intense itch can disrupt sleep, impairing performance at work or school [34], while the altering of early tactile development in infants with AD can negatively impact physical and emotional development [35].

3. Topical Options for the Management of Chronic Pruritus

Topical corticosteroids are the recommended first-line treatment option for the management of AD and have been for over half a century [36,37]. Their exact mechanisms of action, like their potency, vary greatly, but all are intended for treatment of steroid-responsive dermatoses such as AD and psoriasis. The least potent, but most widely used, corticosteroid is hydrocortisone. The efficacy of topical corticosteroids in the treatment of AD is well known, but less well known are their benefits specifically in combating the itch associated with AD. A 1988 study by Wahlgren and colleagues developed a method for recording subjective scoring of pruritus in AD patients treated with the potent topical corticosteroid betamethasone dipropionate versus placebo control [38]. They found that itch intensity was significantly lower during corticosteroid treatment, and the onset of the antipruritic effect was rapid, with a statistically significant difference in pruritus between the groups reached within 24 h [38]. A four-week, double-blind randomized clinical trial in 1998 by Maloney et al. compared the weakly potent clobetasol propionate to its vehicle in the treatment of moderate to severe AD [39]. Three symptoms of AD were assessed: pruritus, erythema and induration/papulation. By Day 4, pruritus had significantly improved in patients receiving clobetasol propionate compared with vehicle [39]. Together, these studies show the potential for topical corticosteroids, even weakly potent ones, in the management of chronic itch.

However, topical corticosteroid use does come with risks for the patient. Generally speaking, the more potent the corticosteroid, the greater the risk of adverse effects such as thinning of the skin, folliculitis, impetigo, telangiectasia and atrophy, and, in rarer instances, herpetic infections and adrenal suppression [40,41]. Another drawback of topical corticosteroid use is the potential for tachyphylaxis, a phenomenon whereby continued use of the product results in diminished effects over time [42]. As the products are self-administered, it is conceivable that patients may then start using more of the product in the notion that it will make up for the diminished effects, thereby increasing the likelihood of adverse events. For these reasons, topical corticosteroid use is only ever for short- to medium-term treatment of AD and other similar conditions, an unsatisfactory approach for the management of pruritus, which needs to be persistent.

Other topical options exist for the treatment of chronic pruritus. Topical calcineurin inhibitors such as tacrolimus and pimecrolimus are frequently used as alternatives to topical corticosteroids for the treatment of AD, yet a 2016 systematic review by Broeders and colleagues found that, while topical calcineurin inhibitors display similar efficacy to topical corticosteroids in treating AD, they were associated with both higher costs and greater adverse events, including burning sensation and pruritus [43]. Due to the importance of histamine in the itch response, topical antihistamines may be of benefit in the treatment of chronic cutaneous itch. However, while topical antihistamines have been found to be effective in treating ocular allergy [44], their effects in treating pruritus of the skin are mixed, and are usually limited in design or inconsistent in findings [45]. Topical doxepin, a potent H1 and H2 receptor antagonist and the only topical antihistamine shown to significantly relieve pruritus in patients with AD, is associated with significant side effects, including allergic contact dermatitis and drowsiness due to systemic absorption [46]. Additionally, due to evidence that the itch in AD is histamine-independent [16], topical antihistamines would have limited to no efficacy in treating AD-related pruritus. Topical capsaicin, or chili pepper extract, has been reported to be an efficacious treatment for itch [47], yet a recent study found that topical capsaicin can actually enhance chronic pruritus, possibly due to the upregulation of Transient Receptor Vanilloid 1-expressing sensory neurons seen in chronic pruritus conditions [48]. Topical anesthetics such as lidocaine and prilocaine are known to have topical anti-pruritic effects by stabilizing sensory fibers and blocking the itch sensation. However, side effects can include allergic contact dermatitis, paresthesia and methemoglobinemia, necessitating the avoidance of these topical agents in children, pregnant women and patients taking oxidizing drugs [49].

Due to the limitations of the treatment options detailed above, there is a need for effective management strategies for chronic itch that encompass topical products that are efficacious but that can also be used indefinitely without the risk of adverse events. One approach would be the use of products designed to support and promote the healthy functioning of the stratum corneum, principally the lipid bilayer and its crucial components: ceramides, cholesterol and free fatty acids.

4. The Key Lipids of the Stratum Corneum and Their Role in Maintaining a Healthy Barrier

4.1. The Chemistry of Ceramides, Cholesterol and Free Fatty Acids

Ceramides are simple sphingolipids formed from a combination of two hydrophobic chains: a sphingoid base and a fatty acid [50] (Figure 1). Within the skin, ceramides are synthesized via three different pathways: de novo synthesis via serine palmitoyltransferase in the endoplasmic reticulum, glucosylceramide degradation by β-glucocerebrosidase, and hydrolysis of sphingomyelin by sphingomyelinase [51]. The stratum corneum contains a complex assortment of ceramide subclasses; early studies utilizing thin layer chromatography identified eight ceramide sub-classes [52], but this has since expanded [53,54] to a total of 15 subclasses when 1-O-acylceramides, a new subclass denoted by the very long acyl chains in the N- and O- positions, is included [55]. Ceramide subclasses are differentiated from each other by their individual sphingoid base group (sphingosine, phytosphingosine, dihydrosphingosine, dihydroxy sphinganine or 6-hydroxysphingosine) and their fatty acid chain (alpha-hydroxy acid, non-hydroxy fatty acid or omega hydroxyl fatty acid) [50]. These ceramide subclasses each contain different species based on their specific combination of fatty acids and base groups, with at least 300 [56] and possibly 1000 [57] distinct species present in the stratum corneum. In terms of the chemistry of the different subclasses, the sphingoid base is usually a long chain amino alcohol of approximately 18 carbon molecules [58], while the fatty acid chain can range from about 24 to 38 carbons in length [59]. Cholesterol is the primary sterol in the lipid bilayer of the stratum corneum. Found ubiquitously in all animal tissues, it plays a crucial role in cell membrane integrity and is derived from the oxidation of the hydrocarbon squalene [60]. It consists of a planar four ring nucleus with a flexible side chain (Figure 1). Free fatty acids are usually saturated, straight, long chain compounds (Figure 1).

4.2. The Ceramides of Note in Atopic Skin

While mechanical disruption to the skin barrier caused by scratching the intense itch associated with AD exacerbates the disease, atopic skin is also deficient in numerous stratum corneum components that play a major role in the healthy functioning of the skin barrier, chief among them being ceramides. Not only are ceramide levels significantly reduced in lesional skin of AD sufferers [61], but reduced levels are also seen in nonlesional skin. Ceramide composition is also markedly different in AD skin compared with normal skin [62], and the ratio of ceramides, free fatty acids and cholesterol can have a profound impact on the skin [63]. Chain lengths of ceramides and free fatty acids in AD skin are also shorter than those found in normal skin, leading to increased permeability of the skin barrier [64]. This decrease in ceramide chain length in AD has been strongly associated with skin barrier disruption, increased transepidermal water loss (TEWL) and greater disease severity [64]. The average ceramide chain length in AD skin has been estimated to decrease by 0.64 ± 0.23 total carbon atoms [65].

Of the 15 different subclasses of ceramides, ceramides 1 and 3 are most strongly associated with AD. Ceramide 1 (EOP) contains a 30-carbon ester-linked fatty acid acylated to sphingosine, while ceramide 3 (NP) contains a 24-carbon fatty acid acylated to phytosphingosine [66] (Figure 3). Ceramide 1, by way of its long chain length that acts as a connector between the lipid bilayers, plays an important role in the organization of lipids in the stratum corneum [67], while ceramide 3 plays a major role in the morphology of the lipid bilayer [68].

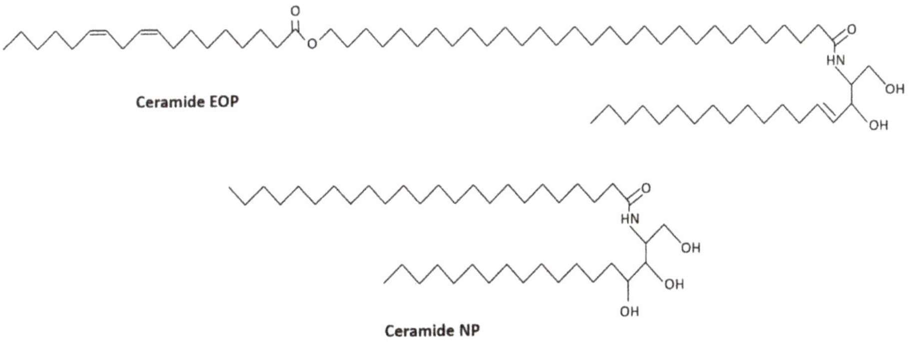

Figure 3. Molecular structures of ceramides EOP and NP. Adapted from [69].

A 1998 study by Di Nardo et al. found that levels of ceramides 1 and 3 were significantly lower in AD skin compared with normal skin, while the level of cholesterol was significantly higher [70]. The ratio of ceramides to cholesterol was also significantly lower in AD patients [70]. The decreased levels of ceramides 1 and 3 was correlated with significantly increased TEWL, a major determinant of dry skin. Similarly, Macheleidt and Sandhoff reported in a 2002 study significantly decreased biosynthesis of ceramides 1 and 3 in both lesional and healthy skin of AD sufferers compared with controls, with the authors concluding that these deficiencies may contribute to the increased permeability of the skin barrier in AD [71].

5. Topical Ceramide Delivery for Itch Relief

If ceramides, particularly ceramides 1 and 3, are significantly reduced in AD skin, it stands to reason that topical delivery of these ceramides may help to restore the skin's barrier function and overcome some of the symptoms of AD, specifically itch. Studies in 1993 and 1995 by Man et al. and Yang et al., respectively, found that the topical delivery of lipids accelerated murine barrier repair after tape stripping and disruption by the solvent acetone [72,73]. While not reflective of AD, the fact that the lipid mixture was able to accelerate repair of a compromised barrier would have obvious benefits for the treatment of AD. Subsequent studies refined the lipids and delivery ratio, and applied them to human skin. A 1996 study by Man and colleagues reported that a mixture of ceramides, free fatty acids and cholesterol delivered topically to human skin accelerated barrier recovery, as evidenced by decreased TEWL [74]. This recovery was dependent on carefully calibrated molar ratios of all three lipids; mixtures with only one or two of the lipids, or an incorrect molar ratio, actually impeded barrier recovery [74]. (The importance of a balanced ratio of all three skin lipids when applied to damaged skin has been detailed in a recent review by Elias et al. [75].) A 2002 study by De Paepe et al. showed that the application of a complete mixture of ceramides, cholesterol and free fatty acid significantly improved barrier recovery 14 days after sodium lauryl sulphate/acetone damage compared with a mixture containing ceramides alone [76]. Berardesca at al. found that an optimized topical skin lipid mixture containing ceramide 3, cholesterol and fatty acids significantly improved multiple parameters, including pruritus, after four and eight weeks of treatment in patients with atopic dermatitis, allergic contact dermatitis or irritant contact dermatitis [77]. In a 2002 Phase 1 trial of a barrier-repair emollient composed of a 3:1:1 molar ratio of ceramides, cholesterol and free fatty acids, the authors reported significant improvements in AD disease severity, TEWL, stratum corneum integrity and skin hydration after treatment [78]. A 2008 study by Huang and Chang found that the topical application of emulsions containing one or both of ceramides 1 and 3 improved the barrier function of skin pretreated with the irritant sodium lauryl sulfate [79]. The authors postulated that ceramides 1 and 3 in combination may act synergistically to decrease TEWL and increase skin hydration [79], an effect that would have great potential in combating dry skin and reducing itch. Chang et al. reported in 2018 that daily application of a formulation containing ceramide and filaggrin, the protein that binds keratin fibers within corneocytes [80], resulted in significant improvements in skin itch, dryness, hydration, desquamation, and overall quality of life of geriatric patients [81]. TEWL improved from baseline but not significantly [81], but this is likely a result of the mechanical nature of aged skin: water content of the skin tends to be lower with age as the skin thins [82]. A 2017 study by Zirwas et al. reported that a single application of a non-prescription moisturizing test material containing ceramides 1, 3 and 6-II and 1% pramoxine hydroxide resulted in a significant reduction in itch severity after 2 min, and showed continued improvement after 8 h [83]. Application of the test material up to four times in a 24 h period for six days resulted in an improvement in itch relief comparable to 1% hydrocortisone [83]. Nearly 90% of participants reported that daily use of the test material over 6 days provided itch relief for the entire night [83].

Topical products containing pseudoceramides and ceramide precursors have also been shown to improve symptoms of AD. Pseudoceramides are synthetic constructs structurally similar to ceramides but with potential differences, such as the lack of a sphingoid base [84]. Draelos and Raymond reported that a cream containing a synthetic ceramide significantly improved skin hydration and skin assessment scores in patients with sensitive skin conditions [85]. Ceramide precursors, such as phytosphingosine, are the less complex foundational parts of the more complex ceramides. A 2013 study found that an emollient containing ceramide precursor lipids improved, among other measurements, pruritus scores in AD patients [86]. While promising, the nature of pseudoceramides and ceramide precursors may make them less efficacious in treating dry skin than ceramides. We previously reported that a topical cream containing a 3:1:1 molar ratio of ceramides (subtypes 1 and 3), cholesterol and free fatty acid (Ego Pharmaceuticals Pty Ltd, Braeside, Victoria, Australia) significantly improved skin hydration and reduced TEWL compared with placebo, with these improvements also being significantly greater than those seen with formulations containing pseudoceramides or ceramide precursors [87].

Ceramide-containing products can also be effective in controlling symptoms of AD other than dry skin and pruritus. A 2018 double-blind, randomized, left-right comparison study by Angelova-Fischer et al. reported that the use of an emollient containing a mixture of ceramide 3, fatty acids, glycerol and licochalcone A significantly reduced the re-occurrence of flares in mild to moderate AD that had been initially cleared by corticosteroid treatment [88]. Corticosteroid treatment was discontinued prior to inclusion in this 12-week study, and the arms treated with placebo experienced significantly worse clinical scoring of atopic dermatitis (SCORAD) and increased TEWL and itch severity [88]. The significant reduction in SCORAD is particularly noteworthy, as the test material used in this study is a non-prescription emollient that can be used indefinitely. Ma et al. reported that a skincare regimen incorporating the twice-daily application of a ceramide-containing moisturizer (and once-daily cleansing with a body wash) both significantly delayed flares and significantly decreased the overall number of flares after 12 weeks in children with a history of mild to moderate AD that had been successfully treated initially with topical corticosteroid [89]. Similar to the study in [88], corticosteroid treatment was discontinued prior to inclusion in the 12-week study. By Week 12, children receiving ceramide-containing moisturizer also had less skin dryness and burning [89]. Similarly, another 2017 study, this one by Koh and colleagues, found that twice-daily use of a ceramide-containing moisturizer for 12 weeks in children with mild to moderate AD significantly improved both carer-assessed patient eczema severity time (PEST), a measure of disease severity made by the sufferer or carer, and clinician-assessed SCORAD [90].

Whether ceramides proper, pseudoceramides or ceramide precursors, the well documented effects of topical ceramide products in increasing skin hydration, decreasing TEWL and improving the severity of flare ups to a degree comparable with corticosteroids make them efficacious, safe [91] and inexpensive adjunct therapies for restoring xerotic skin, but it is the ability to use these products indefinitely that makes them ideal for reducing itch and helping to manage the symptoms of AD.

6. Topical Pine Tar: Itch Relief Millennia in the Making

As described above, first line treatment for AD is the use of topical corticosteroids, but only for short- to medium-term durations. Topical delivery of ingredients found naturally in the skin can help to optimize barrier performance, reducing pruritus indirectly, but is there an active ingredient that can specifically target pruritus therapeutically without the side-effects associated with long-term corticosteroid use? The most effective known ingredient is pine tar. Mass produced topical preparations containing pine tar have been available around the world for over a century, and modern over-the-counter preparations are available in various formulations to help tailor its use to the patient's needs, including gels, lotions and bars [92]. Pine tar, the end product of the destructive distillation of pine wood in extreme temperatures, has been used for centuries for everything from the preservation of ship decking in Scandinavia to its use as a flavoring in the food industry [93]. Its use as a therapeutic agent, however, extends as far back as the age of the father of medicine himself, Hippocrates [94]. Despite this long history of use, the actual mechanism of action and therapeutic activity of pine tar is poorly understood, due simply to the fact that its chemical complexity precludes it from being standardized. As such, its proposed mechanism of action has been extrapolated from studies of coal tar, another commonly-used tar for therapeutic purposes.

What *is* known about pine tar, however, is that it displays potent anti-pruritic and anti-inflammatory properties [95], and is commonly indicated for use in relieving the itch and inflammation associated with numerous chronic itchy skin conditions, including atopic dermatitis and psoriasis [96]. The major benefit of pine tar for the management of chronic itch is its steroid sparing effect; its anti-inflammatory and antipruritic properties reduce itch and the need to scratch, helping to reduce the incidence of AD flare ups while limiting or even eliminating the need for topical corticosteroids. Langeveld-Wildschut et al. treated six patients with 10% pine tar in cetamacrogol ointment, 0.1% triamcinolonacetonide in cetamacrogol ointment or cetamacrogol ointment alone on three separate parts of the back daily for three weeks before patch testing and immunohistochemical analysis of skin biopsies [97]. Pine tar was found to have comparable inhibitory effects to the corticosteroid on the cellular constituents of allergic inflammation, including IL-4$^+$ and CD1+ cells, eosinophils and T-cells [97]. A recent pilot study by Hon et al. compared the efficacy of two complementary bath products, one a pine tar solution (Ego Pharmaceuticals Pty Ltd, Braeside, Victoria, Australia) and the other a preparation containing green tea extract, in the reduction of moderate to severe AD disease severity in children [98]. Daily bathing with the pine tar solution showed significant improvements in, among other parameters, SCORAD, Patient Oriented Eczema Measure (POEM) and Children's Dermatology Life Quality Index (CDLQI) scores after four weeks, each of which measure skin itchiness as the primary symptom [99,100]. The fact that bathing with pine tar can improve AD scoring, coupled with its steroid sparing effect, positions it as an attractive alternative to commonly used treatment strategies for AD such as bleach baths. While studies suggest that bleach baths may be beneficial in the treatment of AD, the nature of bleach baths present many issues. For one, bleach is a household chemical, so is not manufactured to the same level of quality as a therapeutic agent like pine tar. Therapeutic products are subject to strict guidelines covering safety and efficacy data, as well as the requirement to be manufactured according to Good Manufacturing Practice (GMP). Further, the use of bleach baths requires the correct concentration of bleach in water. As a household chemical, there is no standard concentration available. To compound the issue, NaOCl, the active component of bleach, degrades over time so that the concentration of bleach added to baths can vary wildly not only over time but between manufacturers and even different batches of the same product. Adding too much NaOCl to a bath risks irritation and burns for little therapeutic value [101].

The potent anti-pruritic potential of pine tar is bolstered by its safety profile; the minimal phenol content of commercially-available pine tar products means that toxicity is unlikely [96], and, unlike coal tar, pine tar does not cause photosensitization [92]. Crucially, pine tar also does not have the carcinogenic potential that is often attributed to coal tar. A study by Swallow et al. found that a commercially-available pine tar solution (Ego Pharmaceuticals Pty Ltd, Braeside, Victoria, Australia) contained no detectable levels of four of the eight polycyclic aromatic hydrocarbons (PAH) known to cause carcinogenicity in animals [102]. Only minimum detectable levels were found of the other four PAHs, up to 300-fold less than that found in the commercially-available coal tar products [102].

7. Conclusions

Chronic pruritus, and the scratching it necessitates, can have profound physical and psychological effects on sufferers. Given its complex nature, most treatment strategies for chronic itching are unsatisfactory and there is a great need for easily accessible, inexpensive topical options to help manage the urge to scratch. In this review, we provide a brief overview of the pathophysiology of pruritus, its role in atopic dermatitis, and the role the stratum corneum can play in managing the itch. We also briefly discuss the potential of two topically-delivered management options for chronic pruritus: ceramide-dominant emollients and pine tar-based preparations. As adjunct therapies for pruritic skin diseases, the efficacy of both options, especially their steroid-sparing effects, present them as cheap, safe and easily-accessible choices for patients and clinicians that can be used indefinitely without fear of adverse reactions.

Funding: This research received no external funding.

Conflicts of Interest: I.P.H. and F.S. are full-time employees of Ego Pharmaceuticals Pty. Ltd., the manufacturer of the Pinetarsol and QV ranges. The founding sponsors had no role in the design of the study; in the collection, analyses, or interpretation of data; in the writing of the manuscript, and in the decision to publish the results.

References

1. Rothman, S. Physiology of itching. *Physiol. Rev.* **1941**, *21*, 357–381. [CrossRef]
2. Krajnik, M.; Zylicz, Z. Understanding pruritus in systemic disease. *J. Pain Symptom Manage.* **2001**, *21*, 151–168. [CrossRef]
3. Hanifin, J.M.; Rajka, G. Diagnostic features of atopic dermatitis. *Acta Dermatol.* **1980**, *92*, 44–47.
4. Morren, M.A.; Przybilla, B.; Bamelis, M.; Heykants, B.; Reynaers, A.; Degreef, H. Atopic dermatitis: Triggering factors. *J. Am. Acad. Dermatol.* **1994**, *31 Pt 1*, 467–473. [CrossRef]
5. Yosipovitch, G.; Greaves, M.W.; Schmelz, M. Itch. *Lancet* **2003**, *361*, 690–694. [CrossRef]
6. Yosipovitch, G.; David, M. The diagnostic and therapeutic approach to idiopathic generalized pruritus. *Int. J. Dermatol.* **1999**, *38*, 881–887. [CrossRef]
7. Garibyan, L.; Rheingold, C.G.; Lerner, E.A. Understanding the pathophysiology of itch. *Dermatologic* **2013**, *26*, 84–91. [CrossRef]
8. Berger, T.G.; Steinhoff, M. Pruritus and Renal Failure. *Semin. Cutan. Med. Surg.* **2011**, *30*, 99–100. [CrossRef]
9. Hegade, V.S.; Kendrick, S.F.; Rehman, J.; Jones, D.E. Itch and liver: Management in primary care. *Br. J. Gen. Pract.* **2015**, *65*, e418–e420. [CrossRef]
10. Yosipovitch, G.; Samuel, L.S. Neuropathic and psychogenic itch. *Dermatologic* **2008**, *21*, 32–41. [CrossRef]
11. Tivoli, Y.A.; Rubenstein, R.M. Pruritus. *J. Clin. Aesthet. Dermatol.* **2009**, *2*, 30–36.
12. Duan, B.; Cheng, L.; Ma, Q. Spinal Circuits Transmitting Mechanical Pain and Itch. *Neurosci. Bull.* **2018**, *34*, 186–193. [CrossRef]
13. Schmelz, M. Itch and pain. *Dermatol. Ther.* **2005**, *18*, 304–307. [CrossRef]
14. Potenzieri, C.; Undem, B.J. Basic Mechanisms of Itch. *Clin. Exp. Allergy* **2012**, *42*, 8–19. [CrossRef]
15. Urashima, R.; Mihara, M. Cutaneous nerves in atopic dermatitis. A histological, immunohistochemical and electron microscopic study. *Virchows Arch.* **1998**, *432*, 363–370. [CrossRef]
16. Andersen, H.H.; Elberling, J.; Sølvsten, H.; Yosipovitch, G.; Arendt-Nielsen, L. Nonhistaminergic and mechanical itch sensitization in atopic dermatitis. *Pain* **2017**, *158*, 1780–1791. [CrossRef]

17. Hosogi, M.; Schmelz, M.; Miyachi, Y.; Ikoma, A. Bradykinin is a potent pruritogen in atopic dermatitis: A switch from pain to itch. *Pain* **2006**, *126*, 16–23. [CrossRef]
18. Steinhoff, M.; Neisius, U.; Ikoma, A.; Fartasch, M.; Heyer, G.; Skov, P.S.; Schmelz, M. Proteinase-activated receptor-2 mediates itch: A novel pathway for pruritus in human skin. *J. Neurosci.* **2003**, *23*, 6176–6180. [CrossRef]
19. Lee, S.E.; Jeong, S.K.; Lee, S.H. Protease and protease-activated receptor-2 signaling in the pathogenesis of atopic dermatitis. *Yonsei Med. J.* **2010**, *51*, 808–822. [CrossRef]
20. Sonkoly, E.; Muller, A.; Lauerma, A.I.; Pivarcsi, A.; Soto, H.; Kemeny, L.; Steinhoff, M. IL-31: A new link between T cells and pruritus in atopic skin inflammation. *J. Allergy Clin. Immunol.* **2006**, *117*, 411–417. [CrossRef]
21. Lu, J.; Wu, K.; Zeng, Q.; Xiang, Y.; Gao, L.; Huang, J. Serum interleukin-31 level and pruritus in atopic dermatitis: A Meta-analysis. *Zhong Nan Da Xue Xue Bao Yi Xue Ban* **2018**, *43*, 124–130. [PubMed]
22. Matsui, T.; Amagai, M. Dissecting the formation, structure and barrier function of the stratum corneum. *Int. Immunol.* **2015**, *27*, 269–280. [CrossRef] [PubMed]
23. Holbrook, K.A.; Odland, G.F. Regional Differences in the Thickness (Cell Layers) of the Human Stratum Corneum: An Ultrastructural Analysis. *J. Investig. Dermatol.* **1974**, *62*, 415–422. [CrossRef] [PubMed]
24. Harding, C.R. The stratum corneum: Structure and function in health and disease. *Dermatologic* **2004**, *17* (Suppl. S1), 6–15. [CrossRef]
25. Haftek, M. Epidermal barrier disorders and corneodesmosome defects. *Cell Tissue Res.* **2015**, *360*, 483–490. [CrossRef] [PubMed]
26. Avena-Woods, C. Overview of atopic dermatitis. *Am. J. Manag. Care* **2017**, *23* (Suppl. S8), S115–S123.
27. Saito, H. Much atopy about the skin: Genome-wide molecular analysis of atopic eczema. *Int. Arch. Allergy Immunol.* **2005**, *137*, 319–325. [CrossRef]
28. Hanifin, J.M.; Cooper, K.D.; Ho, V.C.; Kang, S.; Krafchik, B.R.; Margolis, D.J. Guidelines of care for atopic dermatitis, developed in accordance with the American Academy of Dermatology (AAD)/American Academy of Dermatology Association "Administrative Regulations for Evidence-Based Clinical Practice Guidelines". *J. Am. Acad. Dermatol.* **2004**, *50*, 391–404. [CrossRef]
29. Werner, Y.; Lindberg, M. Transepidermal water loss in dry and clinically normal skin in patients with atopic dermatitis. *Acta Derm. Venereol.* **1985**, *65*, 102–105. [PubMed]
30. Langan, S.M.; Abuabara, K.; Henrickson, S.E.; Hoffstad, O.; Margolis, D.J. Increased Risk of Cutaneous and Systemic Infections in Atopic Dermatitis—A Cohort Study. *J. Investig. Dermatol.* **2017**, *137*, 1375–1377. [CrossRef]
31. Rinaldi, G. The Itch-Scratch Cycle: A Review of the Mechanisms. *Dermatol. Pract. Concept.* **2019**, *9*, 90–97. [CrossRef]
32. Wahlgren, C.F. Pathophysiology of itching in urticaria and atopic dermatitis. *Allergy* **1992**, *47 Pt 1*, 65–75. [CrossRef]
33. Thyssen, J.P.; Hamann, C.R.; Linneberg, A.; Dantoft, T.M.; Skov, L.; Gislason, G.H.; Egeberg, A. Atopic dermatitis is associated with anxiety, depression, and suicidal ideation, but not with psychiatric hospitalization or suicide. *Allergy* **2018**, *73*, 214–220. [CrossRef] [PubMed]
34. Sibbald, C.; Drucker, A.M. Patient Burden of Atopic Dermatitis. *Dermatol. Clin.* **2017**, *35*, 303–316. [CrossRef] [PubMed]
35. Koblenzer, C.S.; Koblenzer, P.J. Chronic intractable atopic eczema. Its occurrence as a physical sign of impaired parent-child relationships and psychologic developmental arrest: Improvement through parent insight and education. *Arch. Dermatol.* **1988**, *124*, 1673–1677. [CrossRef] [PubMed]
36. Hanifin, J. Atopic Dermatitis: Broadening the Perspective. *J. Am. Acad. Dermatol.* **2004**, 523–524. [CrossRef] [PubMed]
37. Tadicherla, S.; Ross, K.; Shenefelt, P.D.; Fenske, N.A. Topical corticosteroids in dermatology. *J. Drugs Dermatol.* **2009**, *8*, 1093–1105. [PubMed]
38. Wahlgren, C.F.; Hägermark, O.; Bergström, R.; Hedin, B. Evaluation of a new method of assessing pruritus and antipruritic drugs. *Skin Pharmacol. Physiol.* **1988**, *1*, 3–13. [CrossRef]
39. Maloney, J.M.; Morman, M.R.; Stewart, D.M.; Tharp, M.D.; Brown, J.J.; Rajagopalan, R. Clobetasol propionate emollient 0.05% in the treatment of atopic dermatitis. *Int. J. Dermatol.* **1998**, *37*, 142–144. [CrossRef]

40. Gilbertson, E.O.; Spellman, M.C.; Piacquadio, D.J.; Mulford, M.I. Super potent topical corticosteroid use associated with adrenal suppression: Clinical considerations. *J. Am. Acad. Dermatol.* **1998**, *38* (Suppl. S2), 318–321. [CrossRef]
41. Ohman, E.M.; Rogers, S.; Meenan, F.O.; McKenna, T.J. Adrenal Suppression following Low-Dose Topical Clobetasol Propionate. *J. R. Soc. Med.* **1987**, *80*, 422–424. [CrossRef] [PubMed]
42. Du Vivier, A. Tachyphylaxis to topically applied steroids. *Arch. Dermatol.* **1976**, *112*, 1245–1248. [CrossRef] [PubMed]
43. Broeders, J.A.; Ahmed Ali, U.; Fischer, G. Systematic review and meta-analysis of randomized clinical trials (RCTs) comparing topical calcineurin inhibitors with topical corticosteroids for atopic dermatitis: A 15-year experience. *J. Am. Acad. Dermatol.* **2016**, *75*, 410–419. [CrossRef] [PubMed]
44. Ben-Eli, H.; Solomon, A. Topical antihistamines, mast cell stabilizers, and dual-action agents in ocular allergy: Current trends. *Curr. Opin. Allergy Clin. Immunol.* **2018**, *18*, 411–416. [CrossRef] [PubMed]
45. Eschler, D.C.; Klein, P.A. An evidence-based review of the efficacy of topical antihistamines in the relief of pruritus. *J. Drugs Dermatol.* **2010**, *9*, 992–997. [PubMed]
46. Drake, L.; LE, M. The Antipruritic Effect of 5% Doxepin Cream in Patients with Eczematous Dermatitis. *Arch. Dermatol.* **1995**, *131*, 1403–1408. [CrossRef] [PubMed]
47. Anand, P. Capsaicin and menthol in the treatment of itch and pain: Recently cloned receptors provide the key. *Gut* **2003**, *52*, 1233–1235. [CrossRef]
48. Yu, G.; Yang, N.; Li, F.; Chen, M.; Guo, C.J.; Wang, C.; Shi, H. Enhanced itch elicited by capsaicin in a chronic itch model. *Mol. Pain* **2016**, *12*. [CrossRef]
49. Guay, J. Methemoglobinemia related to local anesthetics: A summary of 242 episodes. *Anesth. Analg.* **2009**, *108*, 837–845. [CrossRef]
50. Choi, M.; Maibach, H. Role of Ceramides in Barrier Function of Healthy and Diseased Skin. *Am. J. Clin. Dermatol.* **2005**, *6*, 215–223. [CrossRef]
51. Mizutani, Y.; Mitsutake, S.; Tsuji, K.; Kihara, A.; Igarashi, Y. Ceramide biosynthesis in keratinocyte and its role in skin function. *Biochimie* **2009**, *91*, 784–790. [CrossRef] [PubMed]
52. Elias, P.M.; Brown, B.E.; Fritsch, P.; Goerke, J.; Gray, G.M.; White, R.J. Localization and composition of lipids in neonatal mouse stratum granulosum and stratum corneum. *J. Investig. Dermatol.* **1979**, *73*, 339–348. [CrossRef] [PubMed]
53. Van Smeden, J.; Hoppel, L.; Van der Heijden, R.; Hankemeier, T.; Vreeken, R.J.; Bouwstra, J.A. LC/MS analysis of stratum corneum lipids: Ceramide profiling and discovery. *J. Lipid Res.* **2011**, *52*, 1211–1221. [CrossRef] [PubMed]
54. T'Kindt, R.; Jorge, L.; Dumont, E.; Couturon, P.; David, F.; Sandra, P.; Sandra, K. Profiling and characterizing skin ceramides using reversed-phase liquid chromatography-quadrupole time-of-flight mass spectrometry. *Anal. Chem.* **2012**, *84*, 403–411. [CrossRef] [PubMed]
55. Rabionet, M.; Bayerle, A.; Marsching, C.; Jennemann, R.; Gröne, H.J.; Yildiz, Y.; Sandhoff, R. 1-O-acylceramides are natural components of human and mouse epidermis. *J. Lipid Res.* **2013**, *54*, 3312–3321. [CrossRef] [PubMed]
56. Masukawa, Y.; Narita, H.; Shimizu, E.; Kondo, N.; Sugai, Y.; Oba, T.; Takema, Y. Characterization of overall ceramide species in human stratum corneum. *J. Lipid Res.* **2008**, *49*, 1466–1476. [CrossRef]
57. Moore, D.J.; Rawlings, A.V. The chemistry, function and (patho)physiology of stratum corneum barrier ceramides. *Int. J. Cosmet. Sci.* **2017**, *39*, 366–372. [CrossRef]
58. Vavrova, K.; Kovacik, A.; Opalka, L. Ceramides in the skin barrier. *Eur. Pharm. J.* **2017**, *64*, 28–35. [CrossRef]
59. Breiden, B.; Sandhoff, K. The role of sphingolipid metabolism in cutaneous permeability barrier formation. *Biochim. Biophys. Acta* **2014**, *1841*, 441–452. [CrossRef]
60. Pappas, A. Epidermal surface lipids. *Dermatoendocrinol* **2009**, *1*, 72–76. [CrossRef]
61. Imokawa, G.; Abe, A.; Jin, K.; Higaki, Y.; Kawashima, M.; Hidano, A. Decreased Level of Ceramides in Stratum Corneum of Atopic Dermatitis: An Etiologic Factor in Atopic Dry Skin? *J. Investig. Dermatol.* **1991**, *96*, 523–526. [CrossRef]
62. Ishikawa, J.; Narita, H.; Kondo, N.; Hotta, M.; Takagi, Y.; Masukawa, Y.; Martin, S. Changes in the Ceramide Profile of Atopic Dermatitis Patients. *J. Investig. Dermatol.* **2010**, *130*, 2511–2514. [CrossRef] [PubMed]

63. Joo, K.M.; Hwang, J.H.; Bae, S.; Nahm, D.H.; Park, H.S.; Ye, Y.M.; Lim, K.M. Relationship of ceramide–, and free fatty acid–cholesterol ratios in the stratum corneum with skin barrier function of normal, atopic dermatitis lesional and non-lesional skins. *J. Dermatol. Sci.* **2015**, *77*, 71–74. [CrossRef] [PubMed]
64. Janssens, M.; van Smeden, J.; Gooris, G.S.; Bras, W.; Portale, G.; Caspers, P.J.; Lavrijsen, A.P. Increase in short-chain ceramides correlates with an altered lipid organization and decreased barrier function in atopic eczema patients. *J. Lipid Res.* **2012**, *53*, 2755–2766. [CrossRef] [PubMed]
65. Van Smeden, J.; Janssens, M.; Gooris, G.S.; Bouwstra, J.A. The important role of stratum corneum lipids for the cutaneous barrier function. *Biochim. Biophys. Acta* **2014**, *1841*, 295–313. [CrossRef] [PubMed]
66. Mojumdar, E.H.; Kariman, Z.; van Kerckhove, L.; Gooris, G.S.; Bouwstra, J.A. The role of ceramide chain length distribution on the barrier properties of the skin lipid membranes. *Biochim. Biophys. Acta* **2014**, *1838*, 2473–2483. [CrossRef]
67. Wertz, P.W. Epidermal lipids. *Semin. Dermatol.* **1992**, *11*, 106–113.
68. Engelbrecht, T.N.; Schroeter, A.; Hauß, T.; Demé, B.; Scheidt, H.A.; Huster, D.; Neubert, R.H. The impact of ceramides NP and AP on the nanostructure of stratum corneum lipid bilayer. Part I: Neutron diffraction and 2H NMR studies on multilamellar models based on ceramides with symmetric alkyl chain length distribution. *Soft Matter* **2012**, *8*, 6599–6607. [CrossRef]
69. Robson, K.J.; Stewart, M.E.; Michelsen, S.; Lazo, N.D.; Downing, D.T. 6-Hydroxy-4-sphingenine in human epidermal ceramides. *J. Lipid Res.* **1994**, *35*, 2060–2068. [PubMed]
70. Di Nardo, A.; Wertz, P.; Giannetti, A.; Seidenari, S. Ceramide and cholesterol composition of the skin of patients with atopic dermatitis. *Acta Dermatovenerol. Venereol.* **1998**, *78*, 27–30. [CrossRef]
71. Macheleidt, O.; Sandhoff, K.; Kaiser, H.W. Deficiency of Epidermal Protein-Bound ω-Hydroxyceramides in Atopic Dermatitis. *J. Investig. Dermatol.* **2002**, *119*, 166–173. [CrossRef] [PubMed]
72. Man, M.Q.; Feingold, K.R.; Elias, P.M. Exogenous lipids influence permeability barrier recovery in acetone-treated murine skin. *Arch. Dermatol.* **1993**, *129*, 728–738. [CrossRef] [PubMed]
73. Yang, L.; Mao-Qiang, M.; Taljebini, M.; Elias, P.M.; Feingold, K.R. Topical stratum corneum lipids accelerate barrier repair after tape stripping, solvent treatment and some but not all types of detergent treatment. *Br. J. Dermatol.* **1995**, *133*, 679–685. [CrossRef] [PubMed]
74. Mao-Qiang, M.; Feingold, K.R.; Thornfeldt, C.R.; Elias, P.M. Optimization of Physiological Lipid Mixtures for Barrier Repair. *J. Investig. Dermatol.* **1996**, *106*, 1096–1101. [CrossRef]
75. Elias, P.M.; Wakefield, J.S.; Mao-Qiang, M. Moisturizers versus Current and Next-Generation Barrier Repair Therapy for the Management of Atopic Dermatitis. *SPP* **2019**, *32*, 1–7. [CrossRef] [PubMed]
76. De Paepe, K.; Roseeuw, D.; Rogiers, V. Repair of acetone- and sodium lauryl sulphate-damaged human skin barrier function using topically applied emulsions containing barrier lipids. *J. Eur. Acad. Dermatol. Venereol.* **2002**, *16*, 587–594. [CrossRef] [PubMed]
77. Berardesca, E.; Barbareschi, M.; Veraldi, S.; Pimpinelli, N. Evaluation of efficacy of a skin lipid mixture in patients with irritant contact dermatitis, allergic contact dermatitis or atopic dermatitis: A multicenter study. *Contact Dermat.* **2001**, *45*, 280–285. [CrossRef]
78. Chamlin, S.L.; Kao, J.; Frieden, I.J.; Sheu, M.Y.; Fowler, A.J.; Fluhr, J.W.; Elias, P.M. Ceramide-dominant barrier repair lipids alleviate childhood atopic dermatitis: Changes in barrier function provide a sensitive indicator of disease activity. *J. Am. Acad. Dermatol.* **2002**, *47*, 198–208. [CrossRef]
79. Huang, H.C.; Chang, T.M. Ceramide 1 and ceramide 3 act synergistically on skin hydration and the transepidermal water loss of sodium lauryl sulfate-irritated skin. *Int. J. Dermatol.* **2008**, *47*, 812–819. [CrossRef]
80. Kezic, S.; Jakasa, I. Filaggrin and Skin Barrier Function. *Curr. Probl. Dermatol.* **2016**, *49*, 1–7.
81. Chang, A.L.S.; Chen, S.C.; Osterberg, L.; Brandt, S.; von Grote, E.C.; Meckfessel, M.H. A daily skincare regimen with a unique ceramide and filaggrin formulation rapidly improves chronic xerosis, pruritus, and quality of life in older adults. *Geriatr. Nurs.* **2018**, *39*, 24–28. [CrossRef] [PubMed]
82. Farage, M.A.; Miller, K.W.; Elsner, P.; Maibach, H.I. Characteristics of the Aging Skin. *Adv. Wound Care* **2013**, *2*, 5–10. [CrossRef] [PubMed]
83. Zirwas, M.J.; Barkovic, S. Anti-Pruritic Efficacy of Itch Relief Lotion and Cream in Patients with Atopic History: Comparison with Hydrocortisone Cream. *J. Drugs Dermatol.* **2017**, *16*, 243–247. [PubMed]
84. Meckfessel, M.; Brandt, S. The structure, function, and importance of ceramides in skin and their use as therapeutic agents in skin-care products. *J. Am. Acad. Dermatol.* **2014**, *71*, 177–184. [CrossRef] [PubMed]

85. Draelos, Z.D.; Raymond, I. The Efficacy of a Ceramide-based Cream in Mild-to-moderate Atopic Dermatitis. *J. Clin. Aesthet. Dermatol.* **2018**, *11*, 30–32. [PubMed]
86. Hon, K.; Pong, N.; Wang, S.; Lee, V.; Luk, N.; Leung, T. Acceptability and Efficacy of an Emollient Containing Ceramide-Precursor Lipids and Moisturizing Factors for Atopic Dermatitis in Pediatric Patients. *Drugs R D* **2013**, *13*, 37–42. [CrossRef] [PubMed]
87. Spada, F.; Barnes, T.M.; Greive, K.A. Skin hydration is significantly increased by a cream formulated to mimic the skin's own natural moisturizing systems. *Clin. Cosmet. Investig. Dermatol.* **2018**, *11*, 491–497. [CrossRef] [PubMed]
88. Angelova-Fischer, I.; Rippke, F.; Richter, D.; Filbry, A.; Arrowitz, C.; Weber, T.; Zillikens, D. Stand-alone Emollient Treatment Reduces Flares After Discontinuation of Topical Steroid Treatment in Atopic Dermatitis: A Double-blind, Randomized, Vehicle-controlled, Left-right Comparison Study. *Acta Derm. Venerol.* **2018**, *98*, 517–523. [CrossRef] [PubMed]
89. Ma, L.; Li, P.; Tang, J.; Guo, Y.; Shen, C.; Chang, J.; Kerrouche, N. Prolonging Time to Flare in Pediatric Atopic Dermatitis: A Randomized, Investigator-Blinded, Controlled, Multicenter Clinical Study of a Ceramide-Containing Moisturizer. *Adv. Ther.* **2017**, *34*, 2601–2611. [CrossRef]
90. Koh, M.J.A.; Giam, Y.C.; Liew, H.M.; Foong, A.Y.W.; Chong, J.H.; Wong, S.M.Y.; Cork, M.J. Comparison of the Simple Patient-Centric Atopic Dermatitis Scoring System PEST with SCORAD in Young Children Using a Ceramide Dominant Therapeutic Moisturizer. *Dermatol. Ther.* **2017**, *7*, 383–393. [CrossRef]
91. Choi, S.M.; Lee, B.M. Safety and risk assessment of ceramide 3 in cosmetic products. *Food Chem. Toxicol.* **2015**, *84*, 8–17. [CrossRef] [PubMed]
92. Barnes, T.; Greive, K. Topical pine tar: History, properties and use as a treatment for common skin conditions. *Australas. J. Dermatol.* **2017**, *58*, 80–85. [CrossRef] [PubMed]
93. Allen, L. Basics of Compounding with Tars. *Int. J. Pharm. Compd.* **2013**, *17*, 400–411. [PubMed]
94. Paghdal, K.V.; Schwartz, R.A. Topical tar: Back to the future. *J. Am. Acad. Dermatol.* **2009**, *11*, 294–302. [CrossRef] [PubMed]
95. Braun-Falco, O.; Plewig, G.; Wolff, H.H.; Winkelmann, R.K. (Eds.) *Dermatology*; Springer: Berlin, Germany, 1991; pp. 1149–1150.
96. Schmid, M.H.; Korting, H.C. Coal Tar, Pine Tar and Sulfonated Shale Oil Preparations: Comparative Activity, Efficacy and Safety. *Dermatology* **1996**, *193*, 1–5. [CrossRef] [PubMed]
97. Langeveld-Wildschut, E.G.; Riedl, H.; Thepen, T.; Biharia, I.C.; Bruijnzeel, P.L. Modulation of the atopy patch test reaction by topical corticosteroids and tar. *J. Allery Clin. Immunol.* **2000**, *106*, 738–743. [CrossRef]
98. Hon, K.L.; Ng, W.G.G.; Kung, J.S.C.; Leung, P.C.; Leung, T.F. Pilot Studies on Two Complementary Bath Products for Atopic Dermatitis Children: Pine-Tar and Tea. *Medicines* **2019**, *6*, 8. [CrossRef] [PubMed]
99. Charman, C.R.; Venn, A.J.; Williams, H.C. The patient-oriented eczema measure: Development and initial validation of a new tool for measuring atopic eczema severity from the patients' perspective. *Arch. Dermatol.* **2004**, *140*, 1513–1519. [CrossRef] [PubMed]
100. Lewis-Jones, M.S.; Finlay, A.Y. The Children's Dermatology Life Quality Index (CDLQI): Initial validation and practical use. *Br. J. Dermatol.* **1995**, *132*, 942–949. [CrossRef] [PubMed]
101. Barnes, T.M.; Greive, K.A. Use of bleach baths for the treatment of infected atopic eczema. *Australas. J. Dermatol.* **2013**, *54*, 251–258. [CrossRef] [PubMed]
102. Swallow, W.; Curtis, J. Levels of Polycyclic Aromatic Hydrocarbons in some Coal Tar Skin Preparations. *Aust. J. Dermatol.* **1980**, *21*, 154–157. [CrossRef]

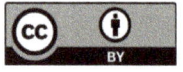

© 2019 by the authors. Licensee MDPI, Basel, Switzerland. This article is an open access article distributed under the terms and conditions of the Creative Commons Attribution (CC BY) license (http://creativecommons.org/licenses/by/4.0/).

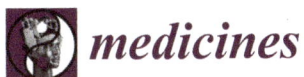

Article

Chronic Pruritus Responding to Dupilumab—A Case Series

Lisa L. Zhai [1,2], Kevin T. Savage [3], Connie C. Qiu [1,2,*], Annie Jin [1,2], Rodrigo Valdes-Rodriguez [4] and Nicholas K. Mollanazar [5]

1. Department of Dermatology, Lewis Katz School of Medicine at Temple University, Philadelphia, PA 19140, USA
2. Lewis Katz School of Medicine, Temple University, Philadelphia, PA 19140, USA
3. Drexel University College of Medicine, Philadelphia, PA 19129, USA
4. Department of Dermatology, University of Virginia, Charlottesville, VA 22903, USA
5. Department of Dermatology, Perelman School of Medicine, University of Pennsylvania, Philadelphia, PA 19140, USA
* Correspondence: connie.qiu@temple.edu; Tel.: +215-707-3376; Fax: +215-707-4058

Received: 23 May 2019; Accepted: 26 June 2019; Published: 29 June 2019

Abstract: Background: Chronic pruritus is defined as itch lasting for greater than six weeks. Pruritus is a burdensome manifestation of several internal and external disease states with a significant impact on quality of life. Dupilumab has shown promise in treating a number of conditions including atopic dermatitis (AD) and asthma. Its success in reducing pruritus in AD has generated interest regarding its potential application in other pruritic conditions, such as chronic pruritus of unknown origin, uremic pruritus, and pruigo nodularis. **Methods:** In this retrospective analysis, we present a series of 20 recalcitrant pruritus patients seen at a tertiary center treated with off-label dupilumab at standard AD dosing. **Results:** Dupilumab was successful at reducing itch in all treated patients, leading to complete resolution in 12/20 patients and an overall mean NRSi reduction of 7.55. Dupilumab was well tolerated with no significant adverse effects. **Conclusions:** Our case series suggests dupilumab may be a safe and efficacious therapeutic option in several pruritic conditions and demonstrates the need for further studies to better ascertain its place in the pruritus treatment armamentarium.

Keywords: dupilumab; IL-4; IL-13; pruritus; chronic pruritus of unknown origin; prurigo nodularis; uremic pruritus; lichen planus; eosinophilic dermatosis of hematologic malignancy; chronic pruritus

1. Introduction

Pruritus, the Latin word for itch, is defined as an "unpleasant sensation that elicits the desire or reflex to scratch" [1]. Perhaps unsurprisingly, pruritus is an extremely common complaint. Over an 11-year period in America alone, pruritus accounted for 1% of all physician visits, bringing the 11-year total to a staggering 77 million visits [2]. In comparison, 1.8% of all physician visits in America were for low back pain [2]. Undoubtedly, these numbers underestimate the extent of the true problem, as studies have demonstrated that only half of patients experiencing pruritus will visit a physician for that problem [2–6].

Pruritus is separated into two clinical categories: acute and chronic. Chronic pruritus (CP) is defined as itch lasting more than six weeks, while acute pruritus (AP) is defined as itch lasting less than six weeks [3]. As many clinicians can attest, antihistaminergic treatments fail to provide patients suffering from CP with any meaningful benefits [7]. This anecdotal finding leads to the hypothesis that there must be an additional pathway besides just histaminergic itch. Indeed, pruritus can further be divided into histaminergic and non-histaminergic itch. We now know that the neurophysiologic and neuroanatomical pathways for histaminergic and non-histaminergic itch, while related, are entirely separate and independent from one another [8–10]. The psychosocial burden of CP and its significant negative impact on quality of life are now well understood. Recently, it was reported that the effects of CP are as debilitating as chronic pain [11–14]. Despite all these recent advances in our understanding of CP, the underlying pathophysiologic mechanisms of CP are not fully elucidated and currently, there are no medications that are specifically FDA approved for the treatment of this debilitating disease. Since CP is associated with myriad systemic and primary dermatologic diseases, there likely is not one single cause of CP. Rather, CP is likely caused by a complex interface between skin, keratinocytes, cutaneous nerve fibers, cytokines, pruritogens, and the peripheral and central nervous systems [15].

While there may not be one single cause of CP, the final neuronal pathway that carries the itch signal from the periphery to the central nervous system may be a conserved constant. Recent bench-to-bedside work has implicated the cytokine IL-4 in the neuronal processes that drive CP. In their seminal publication, Oetjen et al., demonstrated: the receptor for IL-4, IL-4Ra, is directly expressed on sensory neurons in both mice and human dorsal root ganglia; that expression of Th2 cytokines (IL-4, IL-13, and IL-31) directly activates sensory dorsal root ganglia neurons; and that ablation of IL-4Ra abated chronic itching in a murine mouse model [16,17]. Taken together, these findings demonstrated that CP, at least in part, is dependent on neuronal IL-4RA signaling. With the aforementioned findings in mind, it was hypothesized that targeting IL-4RA signaling might act to ablate the itch sensation, regardless of the underlying cause of CP.

In 2018, we reported significant reductions in CP in patients with prurigo nodularis using dupilumab, a novel monoclonal IL-4/IL-13 antagonist approved for the treatment of moderate to severe atopic dermatitis (AD) [18]. Dupilumab is a fully human monoclonal IgG antibody that occupies the shared alpha subunit receptor site for IL-4, which blocks the effects of the IL-4 and IL-13 signaling pathway [15]. IL-4 and IL-13 are thought to be key mediators in the chronic pruritus that is the hallmark of (AD), and are key upstream drivers in the Th2 pathways that modulate myriad downstream targets, such as IL-5 and IL-31 [8,19]. Herein, we present a case-series of 20 patients with CP, of various causes, treated off-label in a busy tertiary academic referral center with dupilumab.

2. Report of Cases

We retrospectively reviewed 20 patients that presented to our tertiary referral center with pruritic skin conditions including chronic pruritus of unknown origin (CPUO), eosinophilic dermatosis of hematologic malignancy (EDHM), lichen planus, prurigo nodularis (PN), and uremic pruritus. Only one patient had a known history of AD as a child. All patients failed topical steroids and topical calcineurin inhibitors. Subcutaneous injections of dupilumab (Dupixent; Regeneron-Sanofi) were administered in the standard AD dosing regimen (600 mg induction dose followed by 300 mg every 2 weeks thereafter). Baseline patient-reported numeric rating scale itch intensity (NRSi) was recorded for each patient prior to therapy initiation. At each subsequent visit, patients reported their NRSi. Mean NRSi reduction was calculated for each subject using their baseline NRSi and the NRSi from their last visit while taking dupilumab. Total itch reduction was defined as an NRSi of 0.

2.1. All Patients with Chronic Pruritus (n = 20)

Mean NRSi (SD): 9.00 (1.21)

Mean NRSi Reduction (SD): 7.55 (2.68)

In total, 20 patients were treated with dupilumab for chronic pruritus (all causes), with between one and five follow up visits (Table 1). Of the 20 patients, 15 had follow-up data at 12 weeks or longer. This cohort demonstrated an initial mean NRSi of 9.00 (SD) (1.21) and a mean NRSi reduction (SD) of 7.55 (2.68) (Table 1 and Figure 1). The trend of response to dupilumab over time can be seen in Figure 2. There was no statistically significant difference with regards to response based on gender. Meaningful statistical significance could not be determined in regard to the rapidity of response due to the small sample size and variance in follow-up time intervals.

Table 1. Summary data.

Patient	A	B	C	D	E	F	G	H	I	J	K	L	M	N	O	P	Q	R	S	T
Age	72	65	66	56	62	82	65	57	52	28	71	78	43	64	55	58	55	63	49	67
Sex	F	M	F	F	M	M	F	F	M	F	F	M	F	M	F	F	F	M	M	M
PMHx Atopic Derm	No	No	No	Yes	No	No	No	No	No	No	No	No	No	No	No	No	No	No	No	No
Diagnosis	Prurigo nodularis	Chronic pruritus of unknown origin	Chronic pruritus of unknown origin	Chronic pruritus of unknown origin	Uremic pruritus	Eosinophilic dermatosis of hematologic malignancy	Chronic pruritus of unknown origin	Uremic pruritus	Lichen planus	Prurigo nodularis	Uremic pruritus	Uremic pruritus	Prurigo nodularis	Uremic Pruritus	Prurigo nodularis	Prurigo nodularis	Prurigo nodularis	Prurigo nodularis	Prurigo nodularis	Prurigo nodularis
Initial NRSi	9/10	9/10	7/10	10/10	8/10	6/10	9/10	10/10	9/10	9/10	10/10	10/10	10/10	10/10	8/10	10/10	10/10	7/10	9/10	10/10
2-week follow-up NRSi	-	-	3/10	-	7/10	4/10	3/10	6/10	7/10	7/10	4/10	7/10	-	3/10	-	-	-	4/10	0/10	-
4-week follow-up NRSi	-	-	0/10*	1/10*	7/10	0/10	-	6/10	1/10	6/10	-	5/10	0/10	0/10	5/10	-	3/10	0/10	-	5/10
8-week follow-up NRSi	0/10*	-	-	-	-	0/10	2/10	5/10	1/10	-	-	5/10	0/10	-	-	-	1/10	-	-	0/10
12-week follow-up NRSi	0/10	-	-	-	-	0/10	1/10	4/10	-	-	1/10	4/10	-	0/10	-	3/10	0/10	0/10	-	0/10
16-week follow-up NRSi	-	-	-	0/10	-	-	-	-	-	-	-	-	-	-	-	-	-	-	-	-
20-week follow-up NRSi	0/10	-	-	-	-	-	-	-	-	-	-	-	0/10	0/10	-	0/10	0/10	0/10	-	0/10
24-week follow-up NRSi	-	1/10	-	0/10	-	-	-	-	-	-	-	-	-	-	-	0/10	-	-	-	-
28-week follow-up NRSi	-	-	0/10	-	-	-	-	-	-	-	-	-	-	-	-	-	-	-	-	-
32-week follow-up NRSi	-	-	-	-	-	-	-	-	-	-	-	-	-	-	-	-	-	-	-	-
36-week follow-up NRSi	-	-	-	-	-	-	-	-	-	-	-	-	-	-	-	0/10	0/10	-	-	-
40-week follow-up NRSi	-	-	-	-	-	-	-	-	-	-	-	-	-	-	-	-	-	-	-	-
44-week follow-up NRSi	-	-	-	-	-	-	-	-	-	-	-	-	-	-	-	0/10	-	-	-	-
48-week follow-up NRSi	-	-	-	-	-	-	-	-	-	-	-	-	-	-	-	-	-	-	-	-
52-week follow-up NRSi	-	-	-	-	-	-	-	-	-	-	-	-	-	-	-	-	0/10	-	-	-
>1 year follow-up NRSi	-	0/10	-	-	-	-	-	-	-	-	-	-	-	-	-	0/10	-	-	-	-
NRSi Reduction	9	9	7	10	1	6	8	6	8	3	9	6	10	10	3	10	10	7	9	10
Total Patients	20																			
Mean Initial NRSi (SD)	9 (1.21)																			
Mean NRSi Reduction (SD)	7.55 (2.68)																			

* Discontinued treatment following this visit due to continued pruritus relief.

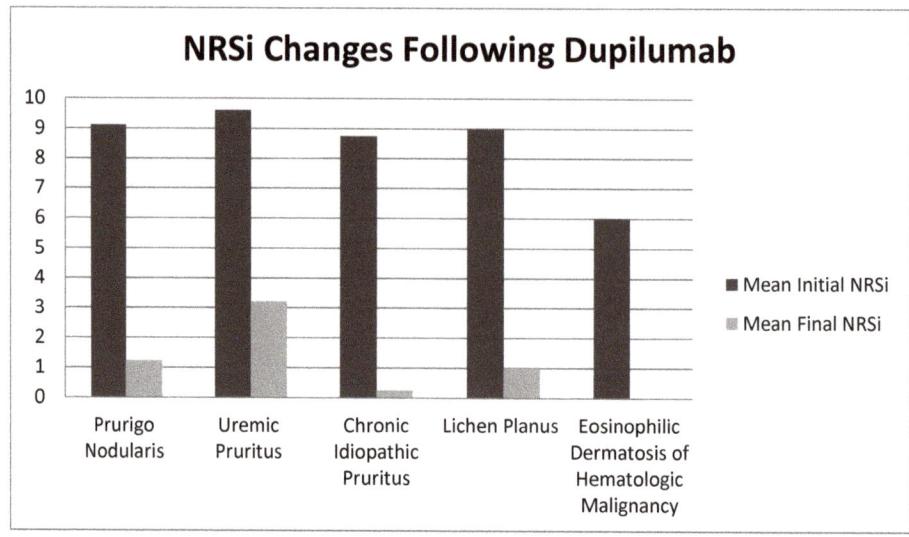

Figure 1. Numeric rating scale itch intensity (NRSi) changes following dupilumab.

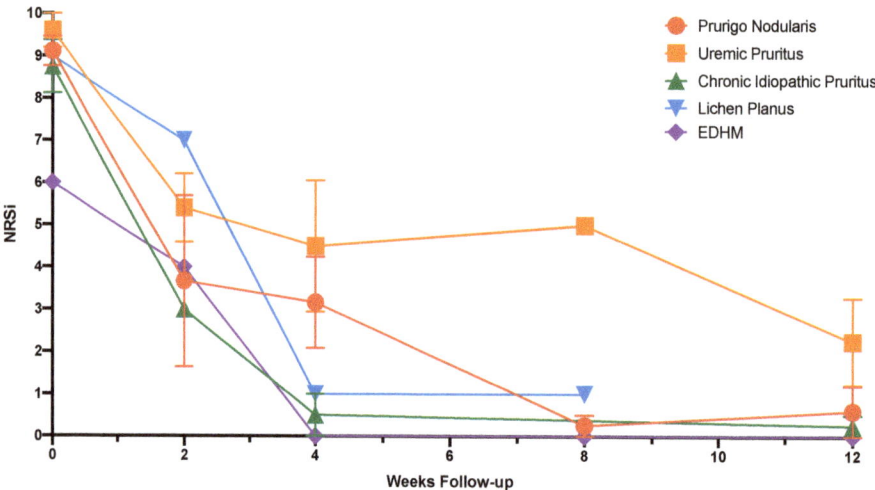

Figure 2. Response to dupilumab by disease over time.

2.2. Prurigo Nodularis (n = 9)

Mean Baseline NRSi (SD): 9.11 (1.05)
Mean NRSi Reduction (SD): 7.89 (2.93)

Nine patients with PN had an initial mean NRSi (SD) of 9.11 (1.05) (Table 2), with between one to five follow-up visits. Of the nine patients, six had follow-up data at 20 weeks or longer. This cohort demonstrated a mean NRSi reduction (SD) of 7.89 (2.93). One patient (denoted with * in Table 2) responded so well that at 8-week follow-up, they elected to go off treatment and remained itch free at 20-week follow-up off treatment.

Table 2. Prurigo nodularis.

Patient	A	J	M	O	P	Q	R	S	T
Age	72	28	43	55	58	55	63	49	67
PMHx Atopic Derm	No	No	No	No	No	No	No	No	No
Diagnosis	Prurigo nodularis	Prurigo nodularis	Prurigo nodularis	Prurigo nodularis	Prurigo nodularis	Prurigo nodularis	Prurigo nodularis	Prurigo nodularis	Prurigo nodularis
Initial NRSi	9/10	9/10	10/10	8/10	10/10	10/10	7/10	9/10	10/10
2-week follow-up NRSi	-	7/10	-	-	-	-	4/10	0/10	-
4-week follow-up NRSi	-	6/10	0/10	5/10	-	3/10	0/10	-	5/10
8-week follow-up NRSi	0/10	-	0/10	-	-	1/10	-	-	0/10
12-week follow-up NRSi	0/10*	-	-	-	3/10	0/10	0/10	-	0/10
16-week follow-up NRSi	-	-	-	-	-	-	-	-	-
20-week follow-up NRSi	0/10	-	0/10	-	0/10	0/10	0/10	-	0/10
>28 week follow-up NRSi	-	-	-	-	0/10	0/10	-	-	-
NRSi Reduction	9	3	10	8	10	10	7	9	10
Total patients					9				
Mean Initial NRSi (SD)					9.11 (1.05)				
Mean NRSi Reduction (SD)					7.89 (2.93)				

* Discontinued treatment after 8 week follow-up visit due to continued pruritus relief.

2.3. Uremic Pruritis (n = 5)

Mean Baseline NRSi (SD): 9.60 (0.89)
Mean NRSi Reduction (SD): 6.40 (3.51)

Five patients with uremic pruritus had an initial mean NRSi (SD) of 9.60 (0.89) (Table 3), with between three to five follow-up visits. Of the five patients, four had follow-up data at 12 weeks. This cohort demonstrated a mean NRSi reduction (SD) of 6.40 (3.51). One patient was hemodialysis dependent while the other patients were not.

Table 3. Uremic pruritus.

Patient	E	H	K	L	N
Age	62	57	71	78	64
PMHx Atopic Derm	No	No	No	No	No
Diagnosis	Uremic pruritis	Uremic pruritis	Uremic pruritis	Uremic pruritis	Uremic Pruritus
Initial NRSi	8/10	10/10	10/10	10/10	10/10
2-week follow-up NRSi	7/10	6/10	4/10	7/10	3/10
4-week follow-up NRSi	7/10	6/10	-	5/10	0/10
8-week follow-up NRSi	-	5/10	-	5/10	-
12-week follow-up NRSi	-	4/10	1/10	4/10	0/10
NRSi Reduction	1	6	9	6	10
Total patients			5		
Mean Initial NRSi (SD)			9.6 (0.89)		
Mean NRSi Reduction (SD)			6.4 (3.51)		

2.4. Chronic Idiopathic Pruritis (n = 4)

Mean Baseline NRSi (SD): 8.75 (1.26)
Mean NRSi Reduction (SD): 8.5 (1.29)

Four patients with CPUO had an initial mean NRSi (SD) of 8.75 (1.26) (Table 4) All four patients had follow-up data at 12 weeks or greater. This cohort demonstrated a mean NRSi reduction (SD) of 8.50 (1.29) (Table 4). Two patients (denoted by * in Table 4) responded so well that they elected to go off treatment at their 4-week follow-up and remained itch free at 20-week follow-up or greater.

Table 4. Chronic pruritus of unknown origin.

Patient	B	C	D	G
Age	65	66	56	65
PMHx Atopic Derm	No	No	Yes	No
Diagnosis	Chronic pruritus of unknown origin	Chronic pruritus of unknown origin	Chronic pruritus of unknown origin	Chronic pruritus of unknown origin
Initial NRSi	9/10	7/10	10/10	9/10
2-week follow-up NRSi	-	3/10		3/10
4-week follow-up NRSi	-	0/10*	1/10*	-
12-week or > follow-up NRSi	0/10	0/10	0/10	1/10
NRSi Reduction	9	7	10	8
Total patients		4		
Mean Initial NRSi (SD)		8.75 (1.26)		
Mean NRSi Reduction (SD)		8.5 (1.29)		

* Discontinued treatment after 4 week follow-up visit due to continued pruritus relief.

2.5. Lichen Planus (n = 1)

Mean Baseline NRSi: 9.0
Mean NRSi Reduction: 8.0

One patient with LP reported an initial mean NRSi of 9, with 3 follow up visits spanning 8 weeks (Table 1). The patient reported a mean NRSi reduction of 8. The patient had previously failed trials of prednisone and acitretin, as well as topical steroids and topical calcineurin inhibitors. Of note, both the patient's rash and itch were noted to improve substantially on treatment.

2.6. Eosinophilic Dermatosis of Hematologic Malignancy (n = 1)

Mean Baseline NRSi: 6.0
Mean NRSi Reduction: 6.0

One patient with EDHM reported an initial mean NRSi of 6, with 4 follow-up visits spanning 16 weeks (Table 1). Prior to initiation of dupilumab, the patient had more severe pruritus that responded to systemic steroids. After 3 courses of month-long prednisone tapers in as many months, the decision was made to switch the patient to a steroid sparing agent. The patient's hematologist was not comfortable with immunosuppressive medications, such as methotrexate, as the patient was receiving chemotherapy for CLL. In the data reported, the patient used only dupilumab and topical corticosteroids as needed.

3. Discussion

Pruritus is mediated through both histaminergic and non-histaminergic pathways [5]. Histaminergic itch is induced by the histamine pathway while non-histaminergic itch appears to be mediated by proteinase activated receptors [8,15]. Cutaneous sensory nerves originate from dorsal root ganglion and terminate in the dermis or epidermis close in proximity to skin cells such as keratinocytes, Langerhans cells, and fibroblasts [15]. Both histaminergic and non-histaminergic itch signals are relayed to the brain via the spinal thalamic tract (STT), but the two do not converge on the same STT neurons [8]. Brain functional imaging studies show that different brain regions, in addition to a core group of brain structures, are selectively activated depending on the type of itch induced [8]. Thus, the distinction between histaminergic and nonhistaminergic itch is seen throughout transmission of the itch signal from the distal periphery to the cortex. This distinction between the two itch pathways explains the clinical quagmire that has vexed physicians for the past several decades regarding the treatment of non-histaminergic itch—traditional anti-histaminergic mediated therapies simply do not work in these patients. All treatments used by clinicians, including commonly used modalities such as phototherapy, are entirely off-label, based on limited case reports, and often carry significant risks. The recent successful report of a Phase 2 clinical trial for Serlopitant (Menlo Therapeutics, Redwood City, CA), a selective NK_1R antagonist, in the treatment of CP is promising and a step in the right direction [17,20]. Nevertheless, there remains an unmet need regarding additional therapeutic agents for the treatment of CP in clinical practice.

We present quantitative data regarding itch intensities and respective reductions from baseline in 20 patients with chronic pruritus. Our mean NRSi of 9.00 is substantially higher when compared to previously reported itch intensities [20]. Most likely, our reported mean itch intensity is significantly higher than previous reports as this cohort represents only patients with severe and substantial disease, which necessitated off-label use of a systemic medication. We report an overall mean NRSi reduction (SD) of 7.55 (2.68), which is on the higher end of previous reports [20]. The higher degree of response reported by our patients in this case series may indicate that dupilumab is effective at abolishing the itch sensation, regardless of the underlying cause. The response to dupilumab in our cohort may be explained by recent bench-to-bedside work, wherein IL-4Ra was found to be expressed directly on sensory neurons in both mice and human dorsal root ganglia [16]. Blockade of the IL-4ra signaling with dupilumab may block neuronal transmission of the itch signal from the periphery to the CNS.

3.1. Prurigo Nodularis

PN was the single largest etiology of CPUO in our cohort (n = 9). The exact prevalence of PN is unknown, though PN is more prevalent in the elderly and in patients with atopy [21]. PN is associated with numerous comorbidities including HIV, cardiovascular disease, and psychiatric illness [22]. Itch from PN is particularly bothersome; in a tertiary itch center, PN patients experienced the worst initial itch intensities and responded the least to treatment [17]. Our patients reported a mean NRSi of 9.11, which is in line from previous reported itch intensities in PN [20].

Although PN pathogenesis is incompletely understood, tryptase, IL-31, prostaglandins, and neuropeptides have all been implicated [23,24]. IL-31 mRNA is markedly elevated in lesional dermis compared to healthy skin [25]. PN patients demonstrate characteristic dermal hypersensitivity resultant from neuronal hyperplasia in the dermis [26]. In the epidermis, however, the opposite is true as there is neuronal hypoplasia, and healed prurigo nodules may demonstrate increased nerve fiber density [27]. Successful treatment of PN with dupilumab has been reported in the literature [18,28,29]. There is evidence to suggest that PN is a Th2 cytokine dependent process, as epidermal biopsies of lesional skin in PN patients show higher levels of STAT6 compared to controls [30]. Importantly, STAT6 is activated in part by IL-4/IL-13 [30].

Neuropeptides also appear to play a role in PN development as PN patients demonstrate an increased number of substance P (SP)-dependent nerve fibers in the skin [31]. SP is a neuropeptide released by activated sensory neurons in the skin and appears to be an important modulator for non-histaminergic itch [32,33]. Substance P binds neurokinin 1 receptor (NK_1R) present on mast cells leading to release of pro-pruritic mediators [15]. NK_1R is involved in modulating SP signaling. Serlopitant has shown promise in PN treatment [34,35]. In a randomized clinical trial of serlopitant vs placebo for PN treatment, serlopitant, a selective NK_1R antagonist, provided a significantly better reduction in NSRi versus placebo through eight weeks of treatment [35]. However, treatment-emergent adverse events were experienced by nearly 75% of patients in the treatment arm, suggesting that serlopitant therapy is not without its drawbacks. Additionally, pregabalin, a neuroleptic, has shown promise in treating PN, illustrating statistically significant decreases in mean itch VAS scores among 30 patients [35–37].

Dupilumab was highly effective at relieving itch in the nine PN patients presented in this series. Despite demonstrating a high mean initial NRSi (9.11), all saw a reduction in itch, with most completely resolving (n = 7) and a mean NRSi reduction (SD) of 7.89. These results are encouraging, as patients treated with more traditional therapies including betamethasone [38] (mean NRSi reduction: 4.9) and pimecrolimus [39] (mean NRSi reduction: 2.7) saw markedly lower mean reductions. More potent immunotherapies including cyclosporine and thalidomide may be efficacious; however, they carry significant risks [40–42]. Our mean NRSi reductions are higher than previous reports from a tertiary itch center, but slightly lower compared to more recent reports on dupilumab in the treatment of PN (mean NRSi reduction: 8.8). Our slightly lower reduction might be due to the fact that we have over double the number of patients previously reported. The rapid and profound response noted in our patients further implicates IL-4/IL-13 in the pathophysiology of PN. Of note, no adverse events were experienced by our nine patients, a striking difference when compared to serlopitant. Randomized controlled trials in PN using dupilumab are needed.

3.2. Chronic Pruritus of Unknown Origin

Chronic pruritus of unknown origin (CPUO) is a devastating and burdensome pruritic condition. CPUO disproportionally affects the elderly, consistent with data from our cohort (n = 4, average age = 63 years) [43]. An underlying immune dysregulation is suspected in CPUO development and maintenance; a study of four elderly patients with CPUO showed marked eosinophilia and IgE levels in biopsies of affected skin [44], consistent with a skewed Th2 immune response. IL-4's interaction with lymphocytes and resident myelocytes—in conjunction with IL-13—are important drivers of Th2 mediated disease states [45]. Additionally, age-related loss of protective Th1 immune cells may hasten the Th2 immune response that is characteristic of this condition [46]. CPUO treatment has traditionally revolved around antihistamine and more recently, anti-IgE therapies, with limited effect [47]. Dupilmab, however, has shown efficacy in treating a wide array of Th2 dependent diseases including AD and asthma, likely through modulation of IL-4 and IL-13's interaction with immune cells [48–50].

The mean initial NRSi of our cohort with CPUO was 8.75, which is not dissimilar from previous reports from a tertiary itch center (NRSi: 8.2). Dupilumab effectively treated itch in all our patients suffering from CPUO, with a mean NRSi reduction (SD) of 8.50 (1.29), which is significantly greater when compared to previous reports showing a mean NRSi reduction of 2.8 [17]. No adverse effects were reported in this cohort.

Dupilumab offered encouraging results in treating CPUO, but it is far from the only treatment used in managing this condition. Naltrexone, a partial antagonist of μ, κ, and δ opioid receptors has demonstrated efficacy in CP treatment as well [51]. Naltrexone exerts its anti-pruritic effect by directly binding opioid receptors in the skin, blocking mast cell, basophil, and IgE-mediated histamine release [52]. Among patients with pruritus caused by underlying systemic disease, 50 mg naltrexone daily resulted in a significant therapeutic response in 70% of patients in just one week, suggesting rapid onset of efficacy [53]. A systematic review of naltrexone use in chronic inflammatory dermatologic conditions found that both high and low dose naltrexone may be efficacious in treating pruritic disease [52]. Naltrexone is a promising new therapy in the treatment of CP. Both naltrexone and dupilumab warrant further controlled trials in the treatment of CPUO.

3.3. Lichen Planus

Lichen Planus (LP) is a cell-mediated immune response of unknown origin that may affect the skin, oral cavity, nails, scalp, genitalia, or esophagus. LP classically presents with pruritic, polygonal, violaceous, flat-topped papules and plaques [54]. LP may be self-limiting and resolve spontaneously within two years. Topical corticosteroids are first-line therapy for all forms of LP, including cutaneous, genital, and mucosal erosive lesions. Systemic therapy with acitretin or an oral immunosuppressant should be considered for patients with severe LP that does not respond to topical treatment [55]. Pruritus is a common complaint by patients with LP, with one study of 30 patients reporting a prevalence of 96.7% [56]. Pruritus is an important and burdensome symptom of LP that is largely unstudied. Pathogenesis of itch in LP has not been fully elucidated, and there are no effective therapeutic modalities alleviating pruritus in patients suffering from this disease [57]. What little literature does exist on the pathophysiology of LP is largely focused on oral manifestations of the disease. When compared to healthy controls, patients with LP have elevated levels of IL-6 in their serum [58]. Furthermore, IL-6 levels correlate with LP disease severity and have been suggested as a possible surrogate marker for disease activity [59,60]. IL-6 is implicated in promoting IL-4 induced Th2 processes and in inhibition of IL-12 induced Th1 pathway [61].

Our LP patient presented with a chronic and severe form of the condition. The patient reported that the associated pruritus caused substantial distress. On dupilumab, our patient experienced improvement in rash and NRSi within one month. The rapidity of improvement and self-reported patient satisfaction indicates that dupilumab may begin to address the unmet need for anti-pruritics in LP.

3.4. Uremic Pruritus

Uremic pruritus (UP), or chronic kidney disease associated pruritus (CKD-aP), is a distressing and frequent symptom in chronic renal failure. UP has been associated with poorer quality of life, and depression [62]. A large, international study estimated the prevalence of moderate to extreme pruritus among patients with end-stage kidney disease on hemodialysis to be 42% [63]. The pathogenesis of UP is not well elucidated, but studies have implicated interleukin-31 (IL-31), which is upregulated by Th2 cells in pruritic disorders such as AD and cutaneous T cell lymphoma [64]. A systemic review of treatments for UP revealed that with the exception of evidence for gabapentin, there remains considerable uncertainty regarding the efficacy of other treatments for UP [65]. Gabapentin is an analog of γ-aminobutyric acid, though it does not interact with γ-aminobutyric acid receptors [66,67]. Gabapentin may modulate itch in the dorsal root ganglion and dorsal horn of the spinal cord by inhibiting the α2δ subunit of voltage-dependent calcium channels, thereby increasing the threshold for neuronal excitation [36,67,68]. Gabapentin significantly reduced itch in hemodialysis patients suffering from UP in a randomized clinical trial, decreasing pruritus scores on a VAS from 8.4 at baseline to 1.2 following treatment. Side effects were limited to dizziness and fatigue, suggesting that gabapentin may be an efficacious anti-pruritic therapy [69,70]. Phototherapy, neuroleptics, antidepressants, and many other treatment modalities are used off-label for UP, each with variable short-term efficacy, limited long-term efficacy, and potential for numerous serious adverse events [71].

Our UP patients all reported improvement in NRSi. Of note, response to dupilumab was slower, and the rate of recurrence was higher than what was observed with other patients in this series. The reasons for this phenomenon are unknown. Perhaps the efficacy of dupilumab is dampened by dialysis, although this would not fully explain the discrepancy in this cohort, as only one patient was HD dependent. Our findings demonstrate the need for further studies regarding the pathophysiology of UP—as treatments may elude us until there is a better understanding of the disease mechanisms.

3.5. Eosinophilic Dermatosis of Hematologic Malignancy (EDHM)

EDHM is a unique eosinophilic skin eruption described in patients with hematologic malignancies that was previously called exaggerated arthropod bite reaction, terminology used in part because the lesions resemble arthropod bites both clinically and histologically [72]. In 2001, Bryd et al. coined the term eosinophilic dermatosis of myeloproliferative disease to refer to eosinophilic eruptions in patients with hematologic disorders [73]. Davis et al noticed a striking resemblance of these lesions to the previously described exaggerated arthropod bites [74]. Notably, their previous study revealed that only 25% of their patients with lesions resembling arthropod bites with prominent eosinophilia had a history of arthropod bites [75]. Accordingly, the lesions were determined to be of the same entity and the term eosinophilic dermatosis of myeloproliferative disease was deemed more accurate [73,74]. As more cases were reported, the term eosinophilic dermatosis of hematologic malignancies became preferred to better encompass the variety of hematologic malignancies associated with the eruption [76–78].

Our EDHM patient presented with an ongoing history of chronic lymphocytic leukemia (CLL), the most commonly associated hematologic malignancy reported with EDHM, although EDHM has been described in the context of acute lymphoblastic leukemia, acute monocytic leukemia, large cell lymphoma, mantle cell lymphoma, and myelofibrosis [76,79]. Previous studies reported that most cases do not respond sufficiently to topical corticosteroids, systemic antihistamines, UV-B phototherapy, or interferon therapy [75]. Several reports have documented partial or complete response to systemic prednisone, which was true for our patient as well [72,80]. Previous studies have also found dapsone to be successful initially, but patients on dapsone had to be discontinued due to side effects [80].

The pathogenesis of EDHM is thought to be due to an imbalance of IL-4 and IL-5, an excess of which is hypothesized to lead to the proliferation of neoplastic B cells considered to be the primary driver of the eruption; importantly, IL-4 is well known to induce B-cell class switching [73,76,78,81,82]. In theory, the mechanism of dupilumab should normalize the excess IL-4, mitigating an instigating factor in the development of the lesions. On dupilumab, our patient experienced a rapid clearing of the rash and a steep improvement of NRSi within two months. The complete and sustained response with the lack of side effects, highlights dupilumab as a possible treatment to fill the unmet need of successful therapeutics in EDHM.

4. Conclusions

Our findings re-capitulate previous reports regarding the success of dupilumab in the treatment of prurigo nodularis and further elaborate on its ability to alleviate pruritus in numerous other itchy dermatoses. Specifically, dupilumab resulted in significant improvement of CP in all 20 patients presented in this series. The magnitude and rapidity of improvement, as well as the absence of significant adverse events further support the need to explore dupilumab as a therapy for CP, ideally in a randomized, controlled fashion.

Author Contributions: Data curation, L.L.Z. and C.C.Q.; Supervision, N.K.M.; Writing—original draft, K.T.S.; Writing—review & editing, A.J. and R.V.-R.

Funding: This research received no external funding.

Conflicts of Interest: Lisa L. Zhai, Kevin T. Savage, Connie C. Qiu, Annie Jin and Rodrigo Valdes-Rodriguez have no conflicts. Nicholas K. Mollanazar reports serving as an investigator in trials sponsored by Sanofi and Regeneron Pharmaceuticals. No other disclosures are reported.

References

1. Ikoma, A.; Steinhoff, M.; Ständer, S.; Yosipovitch, G.; Schmelz, M. The neurobiology of itch. *Nat. Rev. Neurosci.* **2006**, *7*, 535–547. [CrossRef] [PubMed]
2. Shive, M.; Linos, E.; Berger, T.; Wehner, M.; Chren, M.M. Itch as a patient-reported symptom in ambulatory care visits in the United States. *J. Am. Acad. Dermatol.* **2013**, *69*, 550–556. [CrossRef] [PubMed]
3. Mollanazar, N.K.; Koch, S.D.; Yosipovitch, G. Epidemiology of Chronic Pruritus: Where Have We Been and Where Are We Going? *Curr. Dermatol. Rep.* **2015**, *4*, 20–29. [CrossRef]
4. Matterne, U.; Apfelbacher, C.J.; Loerbroks, A.; Schwarzer, T.; Büttner, M.; Ofenloch, R.; Diepgen, T.L.; Weisshaar, E. Prevalence, correlates and characteristics of chronic pruritus: A population-based cross-sectional study. *Acta Derm. Venereol.* **2011**, *91*, 674–679. [CrossRef] [PubMed]
5. Ständer, S.; Schäfer, I.; Phan, N.Q.; Blome, C.; Herberger, K.; Heigel, H.; Augustin, M. Prevalence of chronic pruritus in Germany: Results of a cross-sectional study in a sample working population of 11,730. *Dermatology* **2010**, *221*, 229–235. [CrossRef] [PubMed]
6. Wolkenstein, P.; Grob, J.J.; Bastuji-Garin, S.; Ruszczynski, S.; Roujeau, J.-C.; Revuz, J. French people and skin diseases: Results of a survey using a representative sample. *Arch. Dermatol.* **2003**, *139*, 1614–1619; discussion 1619. [CrossRef] [PubMed]
7. Ständer, S.; Weisshaar, E.; Mettang, T.; Szepietowski, J.C.; Carstens, E.; Ikoma, A.; Bergasa, N.; Gieler, U.; Misery, L.; Wallengren, J.; et al. Clinical classification of itch: A position paper of the International Forum for the Study of Itch. *Acta Derm. Venereol.* **2007**, *87*, 291–294. [CrossRef] [PubMed]
8. Papoiu, A.D.; Coghill, R.C.; Kraft, R.A.; Wang, H.; Yosipovitch, G. A tale of two itches. Common features and notable differences in brain activation evoked by cowhage and histamine induced itch. *Neuroimage* **2012**, *59*, 3611–3623. [CrossRef]
9. Papoiu, A.D.P.; Kraft, R.A.; Coghill, R.C.; Yosipovitch, G. Butorphanol suppression of histamine itch is mediated by nucleus accumbens and septal nuclei: A pharmacological fMRI study. *J. Investig. Dermatol.* **2015**, *135*, 560–568. [CrossRef]
10. Mochizuki, H.; Papoiu, A.D.P.; Yosipovitch, G. Chapter 23 Brain Processing of Itch and Scratching. In *Itch: Mechanisms and Treatment*; Carstens, E.A.T., Ed.; CRC Press/Taylor & Francis: Boca Raton, FL, USA, 2014.
11. Kini, S.P.; DeLong, L.K.; Veledar, E.; McKenzie-Brown, A.M.; Schaufele, M.; Chen, S.C. The impact of pruritus on quality of life: The skin equivalent of pain. *Arch. Dermatol.* **2011**, *147*, 1153–1156. [CrossRef]
12. Zachariae, R.; Zachariae, C.; Ibsen, H.H.; Mortensen, J.T.; Wulf, H.C. Psychological symptoms and quality of life of dermatology outpatients and hospitalized dermatology patients. *Acta Derm. Venereol.* **2004**, *84*, 205–212. [CrossRef] [PubMed]
13. Yosipovitch, G.; Goon, A.; Wee, J.; Chan, Y.H.; Goh, C.L. The prevalence and clinical characteristics of pruritus among patients with extensive psoriasis. *Br. J. Dermatol.* **2000**, *143*, 969–973. [CrossRef]
14. Zachariae, R.; Zachariae, C.O.; Lei, U.; Pedersen, A.F. Affective and sensory dimensions of pruritus severity: Associations with psychological symptoms and quality of life in psoriasis patients. *Acta Derm. Venereol.* **2008**, *88*, 121–127. [CrossRef] [PubMed]
15. Mollanazar, N.K.; Smith, P.K.; Yosipovitch, G. Mediators of Chronic Pruritus in Atopic Dermatitis: Getting the Itch Out? *Clin. Rev. Allergy Immunol.* **2016**, *51*, 263–292. [CrossRef] [PubMed]

16. Oetjen, L.K.; Mack, M.R.; Feng, J.; Whelan, T.M.; Niu, H.; Guo, C.J.; Chen, S.; Trier, A.M.; Xu, A.J.; Tripathi, S.V.; et al. Sensory Neurons Co-opt Classical Immune Signaling Pathways to Mediate Chronic Itch. *Cell* **2017**, *171*, 217–228.e213. [CrossRef] [PubMed]
17. Mollanazar, N.K.; Sethi, M.; Rodriguez, R.V.; Nattkemper, L.A.; Ramsey, F.V.; Zhao, H.; Yosipovitch, G. Retrospective analysis of data from an itch center: Integrating validated tools in the electronic health record. *J. Am. Acad. Dermatol.* **2016**, *75*, 842–844. [CrossRef]
18. Mollanazar, N.K.; Elgash, M.; Weaver, L.; Valdes-Rodriguez, R.; Hsu, S. Reduced itch associated with dupilumab treatment in 4 patients with prurigo nodularis. *JAMA Dermatol.* **2018**. [CrossRef]
19. Trier, A.M.; Kim, B.S. Cytokine modulation of atopic itch. *Curr. Opin. Immunol.* **2018**, *54*, 7–12. [CrossRef]
20. Yosipovitch, G.; Ständer, S.; Kerby, M.B.; Larrick, J.W.; Perlman, A.J.; Schnipper, E.F.; Zhang, X.; Tang, J.Y.; Luger, T.; Steinhoff, M. Serlopitant for the treatment of chronic pruritus: Results of a randomized, multicenter, placebo-controlled phase 2 clinical trial. *J. Am. Acad. Dermatol.* **2018**, *78*, 882–891.e810. [CrossRef]
21. Iking, A.; Grundmann, S.; Chatzigeorgakidis, E.; Phan, N.Q.; Klein, D.; Ständer, S. Prurigo as a symptom of atopic and non-atopic diseases: Aetiological survey in a consecutive cohort of 108 patients. *J. Eur. Acad. Dermatol. Venereol.* **2013**, *27*, 550–557. [CrossRef]
22. Boozalis, E.; Tang, O.; Patel, S.; Semenov, Y.R.; Pereira, M.P.; Stander, S.; Kang, S.; Kwatra, S.G. Ethnic differences and comorbidities of 909 prurigo nodularis patients. *J. Am. Acad. Dermatol.* **2018**, *79*, 714–719.e713. [CrossRef] [PubMed]
23. Johansson, O.; Liang, Y.; Emtestam, L. Increased nerve growth factor- and tyrosine kinase A-like immunoreactivities in prurigo nodularis skin—An exploration of the cause of neurohyperplasia. *Arch. Dermatol. Res.* **2002**, *293*, 614–619. [CrossRef] [PubMed]
24. Groneberg, D.A.; Serowka, F.; Peckenschneider, N.; Artuc, M.; Grützkau, A.; Fischer, A.; Henz, B.M.; Welker, P. Gene expression and regulation of nerve growth factor in atopic dermatitis mast cells and the human mast cell line-1. *J. Neuroimmunol.* **2005**, *161*, 87–92. [CrossRef] [PubMed]
25. Sonkoly, E.; Muller, A.; Lauerma, A.I.; Pivarsi, A.; Soto, H.; Kemeny, L.; Alenius, H.; Dieu-Nosjean, M.C.; Meller, S.; Rieker, J.; et al. IL-31: A new link between T cells and pruritus in atopic skin inflammation. *J. Allergy Clin. Immunol.* **2006**, *117*, 411–417. [CrossRef] [PubMed]
26. Weigelt, N.; Metze, D.; Ständer, S. Prurigo nodularis: Systematic analysis of 58 histological criteria in 136 patients. *J. Cutan Pathol.* **2010**, *37*, 578–586. [CrossRef] [PubMed]
27. Schuhknecht, B.; Marziniak, M.; Wissel, A.; Phan, N.Q.; Pappai, D.; Dangelmaier, J.; Ständer, S. Reduced intraepidermal nerve fibre density in lesional and nonlesional prurigo nodularis skin as a potential sign of subclinical cutaneous neuropathy. *Br. J. Dermatol.* **2011**, *165*, 85–91. [CrossRef]
28. Calugareanu, A.; Jachiet, M.; Lepelletier, C.; Masson, A.D.; Rybojad, M.; Bagot, M.; Bouaziz, J.D. Dramatic improvement of generalized prurigo nodularis with dupilumab. *J. Eur. Acad. Dermatol. Venereol.* **2019**. [CrossRef]
29. Beck, K.M.; Yang, E.J.; Sekhon, S.; Bhutani, T.; Liao, W. Dupilumab Treatment for Generalized Prurigo Nodularis. *JAMA Dermatol.* **2019**, *155*, 118–120. [CrossRef]
30. Fukushi, S.; Yamasaki, K.; Aiba, S. Nuclear localization of activated STAT6 and STAT3 in epidermis of prurigo nodularis. *Br. J. Dermatol.* **2011**, *165*, 990–996. [CrossRef]
31. Haas, S.; Capellino, S.; Phan, N.Q.; Böhm, M.; Luger, T.A.; Straub, R.H.; Ständer, S. Low density of sympathetic nerve fibers relative to substance P-positive nerve fibers in lesional skin of chronic pruritus and prurigo nodularis. *J. Dermatol. Sci.* **2010**, *58*, 193–197. [CrossRef]
32. Steinhoff, M.S.; von Mentzer, B.; Geppetti, P.; Pothoulakis, C.; Bunnett, N.W. Tachykinins and their receptors: Contributions to physiological control and the mechanisms of disease. *Physiol. Rev.* **2014**, *94*, 265–301. [CrossRef] [PubMed]
33. Church, M.K.; Okayama, Y.; el-Lati, S. Mediator secretion from human skin mast cells provoked by immunological and non-immunological stimulation. *Skin. Pharmacol.* **1991**, *4* (Suppl. 1), 15–24. [CrossRef] [PubMed]
34. Frenkl, T.L.; Zhu, H.; Reiss, T.; Seltzer, O.; Rosenberg, E.; Green, S. A multicenter, double-blind, randomized, placebo controlled trial of a neurokinin-1 receptor antagonist for overactive bladder. *J. Urol.* **2010**, *184*, 616–622. [CrossRef] [PubMed]

35. Ständer, S.; Kwon, P.; Hirman, J.; Perlman, A.J.; Weisshaar, E.; Metz, M.; Luger, T.A.; TCP-102 Study Group. Serlopitant reduced pruritus in patients with prurigo nodularis in a phase 2, randomized, placebo-controlled trial. *J. Am. Acad. Dermatol.* **2019**, *80*, 1395–1402. [CrossRef] [PubMed]
36. Matsuda, K.M.; Sharma, D.; Schonfeld, A.R.; Kwatra, S.G. Gabapentin and pregabalin for the treatment of chronic pruritus. *J. Am. Acad. Dermatol.* **2016**, *75*, 619–625.e616. [CrossRef] [PubMed]
37. Mazza, M.; Guerriero, G.; Marano, G.; Janiri, L.; Bria, P.; Mazza, S. Treatment of prurigo nodularis with pregabalin. *J. Clin. Pharm. Ther.* **2013**, *38*, 16–18. [CrossRef] [PubMed]
38. Saraceno, R.; Chiricozzi, A.; Nisticò, S.P.; Tiberti, S.; Chimenti, S. An occlusive dressing containing betamethasone valerate 0.1% for the treatment of prurigo nodularis. *J. Dermatolog. Treat.* **2010**, *21*, 363–366. [CrossRef] [PubMed]
39. Siepmann, D.; Lotts, T.; Blome, C.; Braeutigam, M.; Phan, N.Q.; Butterfass-Bahloul, T.; Augustin, M.; Luger, T.A.; Ständer, S. Evaluation of the antipruritic effects of topical pimecrolimus in non-atopic prurigo nodularis: Results of a randomized, hydrocortisone-controlled, double-blind phase II trial. *Dermatology* **2013**, *227*, 353–360. [CrossRef] [PubMed]
40. Andersen, T.P.; Fogh, K. Thalidomide in 42 patients with prurigo nodularis Hyde. *Dermatology* **2011**, *223*, 107–112. [CrossRef]
41. Siepmann, D.; Luger, T.A.; Ständer, S. Antipruritic effect of cyclosporine microemulsion in prurigo nodularis: Results of a case series. *J. Dtsch. Dermatol. Ges.* **2008**, *6*, 941–946. [CrossRef]
42. Aguh, C.; Kwatra, S.G.; He, A.; Okoye, G.A. Thalidomide for the treatment of chronic refractory prurigo nodularis. *Dermatol. Online J.* **2018**, *24*, 6.
43. Valdes-Rodriguez, R.; Stull, C.; Yosipovitch, G. Chronic pruritus in the elderly: Pathophysiology, diagnosis and management. *Drugs Aging* **2015**, *32*, 201–215. [CrossRef] [PubMed]
44. Xu, A.Z.; Tripathi, S.V.; Kau, A.L.; Schaffer, A.; Kim, B.S. Immune dysregulation underlies a subset of patients with chronic pruritus of unknown origin. *J. Am. Acad. Dermatol.* **2016**, *74*, 1017–1020. [CrossRef] [PubMed]
45. Wills-Karp, M.; Finkelman, F.D. Untangling the complex web of IL-4- and IL-13-mediated signaling pathways. *Sci. Signal.* **2008**, *1*, pe55. [CrossRef] [PubMed]
46. Shevchenko, A.; Valdes-Rodriguez, R.; Yosipovitch, G. Causes, pathophysiology, and treatment of pruritus in the mature patient. *Clin. Dermatol.* **2018**, *36*, 140–151. [CrossRef] [PubMed]
47. Maurer, M.; Rosén, K.; Hsieh, H.J.; Saini, S.; Grattan, C.; Giménez-Arnau, A.; Agarwal, S.; Doyle, R.; Canvin, J.; Kaplan, A.; et al. Omalizumab for the treatment of chronic idiopathic or spontaneous urticaria. *N. Engl. J. Med.* **2013**, *368*, 924–935. [CrossRef] [PubMed]
48. Wenzel, S.; Ford, L.; Pearlman, D.; Spector, S.; Sher, L.; Skobieranda, F.; Wang, L.; Kirkesseli, S.; Rocklin, R.; Bock, B.; et al. Dupilumab in persistent asthma with elevated eosinophil levels. *N. Engl. J. Med.* **2013**, *368*, 2455–2466. [CrossRef]
49. Wenzel, S.; Castro, M.; Corren, J.; Maspero, J.; Wang, L.; Zhang, B.; Pirozzi, G.; Sutherland, E.R.; Evans, R.R.; Joish, V.N.; et al. Dupilumab efficacy and safety in adults with uncontrolled persistent asthma despite use of medium-to-high-dose inhaled corticosteroids plus a long-acting β2 agonist: A randomised double-blind placebo-controlled pivotal phase 2b dose-ranging trial. *Lancet* **2016**, *388*, 31–44. [CrossRef]
50. Blauvelt, A.; de Bruin-Weller, M.; Gooderham, M.; Cather, J.C.; Weisman, J.; Pariser, D.; Simpson, E.L.; Papp, K.A.; Hong, H.C.H.; Rubel, D.; et al. Long-term management of moderate-to-severe atopic dermatitis with dupilumab and concomitant topical corticosteroids (LIBERTY AD CHRONOS): A 1-year, randomised, double-blinded, placebo-controlled, phase 3 trial. *Lancet* **2017**, *389*, 2287–2303. [CrossRef]
51. Bihari, B. Efficacy of low dose naltrexone as an immune stabilizing agent for the treatment of HIV/AIDS. *AIDS Patient Care* **1995**, *9*, 3. [CrossRef]
52. Ekelem, C.; Juhasz, M.; Khera, P.; Mesinkovska, N.A. Utility of Naltrexone Treatment for Chronic Inflammatory Dermatologic Conditions: A Systematic Review. *JAMA Dermatol.* **2019**, *155*, 229–236. [CrossRef] [PubMed]
53. Metze, D.; Reimann, S.; Beissert, S.; Luger, T. Efficacy and safety of naltrexone, an oral opiate receptor antagonist, in the treatment of pruritus in internal and dermatological diseases. *J. Am. Acad. Dermatol.* **1999**, *41*, 533–539. [PubMed]
54. Weston, G.; Payette, M. Update on lichen planus and its clinical variants. *Int. J. Womens Dermatol.* **2015**, *1*, 140–149. [CrossRef] [PubMed]
55. Usatine, R.P.; Tinitigan, M. Diagnosis and treatment of lichen planus. *Am. Fam. Physician* **2011**, *84*, 53–60. [PubMed]

56. Reich, A.; Welz-Kubiak, K.; Szepietowski, J.C. Pruritus differences between psoriasis and lichen planus. *Acta Derm. Venereol.* **2011**, *91*, 605–606. [CrossRef] [PubMed]
57. Welz-Kubiak, K.; Reich, A. Mediators of pruritus in lichen planus. *Autoimmune Dis.* **2013**, *2013*, 941431. [CrossRef] [PubMed]
58. Yin, M.; Li, G.; Song, H.; Lin, S. Identifying the association between interleukin-6 and lichen planus: A meta-analysis. *Biomed. Rep.* **2017**, *6*, 571–575. [CrossRef] [PubMed]
59. Sun, A.; Chia, J.S.; Chang, Y.F.; Chiang, C.P. Serum interleukin-6 level is a useful marker in evaluating therapeutic effects of levamisole and Chinese medicinal herbs on patients with oral lichen planus. *J. Oral. Pathol. Med.* **2002**, *31*, 196–203. [CrossRef] [PubMed]
60. Rhodus, N.L.; Cheng, B.; Bowles, W.; Myers, S.; Miller, L.; Ondrey, F. Proinflammatory cytokine levels in saliva before and after treatment of (erosive) oral lichen planus with dexamethasone. *Oral Dis.* **2006**, *12*, 112–116. [CrossRef] [PubMed]
61. Diehl, S.; Rincón, M. The two faces of IL-6 on Th1/Th2 differentiation. *Mol. Immunol.* **2002**, *39*, 531–536. [CrossRef]
62. Sukul, N.; Speyer, E.; Tu, C.; Bieber, B.A.; Li, Y.; Lopes, A.A.; Asahi, K.; Mariani, L.; Laville, M.; Rayner, H.C.; et al. Pruritus and Patient Reported Outcomes in Non-Dialysis CKD. *Clin. J. Am. Soc. Nephrol.* **2019**. [CrossRef] [PubMed]
63. Pisoni, R.L.; Wikström, B.; Elder, S.J.; Akizawa, T.; Asano, Y.; Keen, N.L.; Saran, R.; Mendelssohn, D.C.; Young, E.W.; Port, F.K. Pruritus in haemodialysis patients: International results from the Dialysis Outcomes and Practice Patterns Study (DOPPS). *Nephrol. Dial. Transplant.* **2006**, *21*, 3495–3505. [CrossRef] [PubMed]
64. Gangemi, S.; Quartuccio, S.; Casciaro, M.; Trapani, G.; Minciullo, P.L.; Imbalzano, E. Interleukin 31 and skin diseases: A systematic review. *Allergy Asthma Proc.* **2017**, *38*, 401–408. [CrossRef] [PubMed]
65. Simonsen, E.; Komenda, P.; Lerner, B.; Askin, N.; Bohm, C.; Shaw, J.; Tangri, N.; Rigatto, C. Treatment of Uremic Pruritus: A Systematic Review. *Am. J. Kidney Dis.* **2017**, *70*, 638–655. [CrossRef] [PubMed]
66. Taylor, C.P.; Gee, N.S.; Su, T.Z.; Kocsis, J.D.; Welty, D.F.; Brown, J.P.; Dooley, D.; Boden, P.; Singh, L. A summary of mechanistic hypotheses of gabapentin pharmacology. *Epilepsy Res.* **1998**, *29*, 233–249. [CrossRef]
67. Li, Z.; Taylor, C.P.; Weber, M.; Piechan, J.; Prior, F.; Bian, F.; Cui, M.; Hoffman, D.; Donevan, S. Pregabalin is a potent and selective ligand for α(2)δ-1 and α(2)δ-2 calcium channel subunits. *Eur. J. Pharmacol.* **2011**, *667*, 80–90. [CrossRef] [PubMed]
68. Quintero, J.E.; Dooley, D.J.; Pomerleau, F.; Huettl, P.; Gerhardt, G.A. Amperometric measurement of glutamate release modulation by gabapentin and pregabalin in rat neocortical slices: Role of voltage-sensitive Ca2+ α2δ-1 subunit. *J. Pharmacol. Exp. Ther.* **2011**, *338*, 240–245. [CrossRef] [PubMed]
69. Gunal, A.I.; Ozalp, G.; Yoldas, T.K.; Gunal, S.Y.; Kirciman, E.; Celiker, H. Gabapentin therapy for pruritus in haemodialysis patients: A randomized, placebo-controlled, double-blind trial. *Nephrol. Dial. Transplant.* **2004**, *19*, 3137–3139. [CrossRef]
70. Naini, A.E.; Harandi, A.A.; Khanbabapour, S.; Shahidi, S.; Seirafiyan, S.; Mohseni, M. Gabapentin: A promising drug for the treatment of uremic pruritus. *Saudi J. Kidney Dis. Transplant.* **2007**, *18*, 378–381.
71. Silverberg, J.I.; Brieva, J. A successful case of dupilumab treatment for severe uremic pruritus. *JAAD Case Rep.* **2019**, *5*, 339–341. [CrossRef]
72. Barzilai, A.; Shpiro, D.; Goldberg, I.; Yacob-Hirsch, Y.; Diaz-Cascajo, C.; Meytes, D.; Schiby, R.; Amariglio, N.; Trau, H. Insect bite-like reaction in patients with hematologic malignant neoplasms. *Arch. Dermatol.* **1999**, *135*, 1503–1507. [CrossRef] [PubMed]
73. Byrd, J.A.; Scherschun, L.; Chaffins, M.L.; Fivenson, D.P. Eosinophilic dermatosis of myeloproliferative disease: Characterization of a unique eruption in patients with hematologic disorders. *Arch. Dermatol.* **2001**, *137*, 1378–1380. [PubMed]
74. Davis, M.D.; McEvoy, M.T. Eosinophilic dermatosis associated with hematologic disorders: Not so unique. *Arch. Dermatol.* **2002**, *138*, 1516. [CrossRef] [PubMed]
75. Davis, M.D.; Perniciaro, C.; Dahl, P.R.; Randle, H.W.; McEvoy, M.T.; Leiferman, K.M. Exaggerated arthropod-bite lesions in patients with chronic lymphocytic leukemia: A clinical, histopathologic, and immunopathologic study of eight patients. *J. Am. Acad. Dermatol.* **1998**, *39*, 27–35. [CrossRef]
76. Farber, M.J.; La Forgia, S.; Sahu, J.; Lee, J.B. Eosinophilic dermatosis of hematologic malignancy. *J. Cutan. Pathol.* **2012**, *39*, 690–695. [CrossRef] [PubMed]

77. Qiao, J.; Sun, C.E.; Zhu, W.; Zhu, D.; Fang, H. Flame figures associated with eosinophilic dermatosis of hematologic malignancy: Is it possible to distinguish the condition from eosinophilic cellulitis in patients with hematoproliferative disease? *Int. J. Clin. Exp. Pathol.* **2013**, *6*, 1683–1687.
78. Bari, O.; Cohen, P.R. Eosinophilic dermatosis of hematologic malignancy mimicking varicella zoster infection: Report in a woman with chronic lymphocytic leukemia and review of the literature. *Dermatol. Pract. Concept.* **2017**, *7*, 6–15. [CrossRef]
79. Penn, L.; Ahern, I.; Mir, A.; Meehan, S.A. Eosinophilic dermatitis of hematologic malignancy. *Dermatol. Online J.* **2015**, *21*, 10.
80. Bairey, O.; Goldschmidt, N.; Ruchlemer, R.; Tadmor, T.; Rahimi-Levene, N.; Yuklea, M.; Shvidel, L.; Berrebi, A.; Polliack, A.; Herishanu, Y.; et al. Insect-bite-like reaction in patients with chronic lymphocytic leukemia: A study from the Israeli Chronic Lymphocytic Leukemia Study Group. *Eur. J. Haematol.* **2012**, *89*, 491–496. [CrossRef]
81. Jayasekera, P.S.; Bakshi, A.; Al-Sharqi, A. Eosinophilic dermatosis of haematological malignancy. *Clin. Exp. Dermatol.* **2016**, *41*, 692–695. [CrossRef]
82. Meiss, F.; Technau-Hafsi, K.; Kern, J.S.; May, A.M. Eosinophilic dermatosis of hematologic malignancy: Correlation of molecular characteristics of skin lesions and extracutaneous manifestations of hematologic malignancy. *J. Cutan. Pathol.* **2019**, *46*, 175–181. [CrossRef] [PubMed]

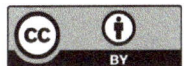

© 2019 by the authors. Licensee MDPI, Basel, Switzerland. This article is an open access article distributed under the terms and conditions of the Creative Commons Attribution (CC BY) license (http://creativecommons.org/licenses/by/4.0/).

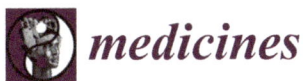

Letter

Mirtazapine for the Treatment of Chronic Pruritus

Raveena Khanna [1,2], Emily Boozalis [1], Micah Belzberg [1], John G. Zampella [3] and Shawn G. Kwatra [1,*]

1. Department of Dermatology, Johns Hopkins University School of Medicine, Baltimore, MD 21231, USA
2. Creighton University School of Medicine, Omaha, NE 68178, USA
3. Department of Dermatology, New York University School of Medicine, New York, NY 10016, USA
* Correspondence: skwatra1@jhmi.edu

Received: 15 June 2019; Accepted: 5 July 2019; Published: 6 July 2019

Abstract: Background: Chronic pruritus is a debilitating condition associated with a wide range of dermatologic, systemic and psychogenic etiologies. In patients with chronic pruritus that is refractory to conventional therapy, symptoms can significantly decrease quality of life by contributing to anxiety, sleep disturbances, and in many cases depression. Recent studies have demonstrated the effectiveness of mirtazapine in relieving chronic itch that is refractory to standard first-line therapies. **Methods:** We searched PubMed for English-language articles containing the words ("pruritus" or "itch") AND "antidepressant" and then conducted a systematic review of the current literature to summarize the efficacy of mirtazapine in treating chronic itch. **Results:** All studies reported a reduction in itch intensity following the administration of mirtazapine. **Conclusion:** Collectively, these studies suggest the potential for mirtazapine to relieve chronic itch attributed to dermatological causes and malignancies. As, such mirtazapine may be an option for patients with chronic pruritus that is refractory to typical first-line treatments.

Keywords: mirtazapine; chronic; pruritus; itch; refractory; treatment; noradrenergic; serotonergic; antihistaminergic; antidepressant

---

Dear Editor,

Chronic pruritus is a common condition that can interfere with sleep and diminish overall quality of life. The current management of chronic itch is directed at the underlying cause, which can be dermatologic, systemic or psychogenic in nature [1]. First-line therapy typically begins with topical emollients, topical corticosteroids, and antihistamines. GABA-receptor modulators, opioid agonists/antagonists and phototherapy can be used for patients with refractory pruritus [1].

Recalcitrant itch is a distressing symptom for which a safe and effective agent is needed [2,3]. Recent studies have demonstrated the effectiveness of oral antidepressants in relieving chronic itch associated with dermatologic, systemic and psychogenic causes [4,5]. Mirtazapine, a dual noradrenergic and serotonergic antidepressant with antihistaminergic properties, is one such antidepressant that has demonstrated effectiveness in reducing itch severity. As an H_1, $5HT_2$ and $5HT_3$-receptor blocker, mirtazapine may be an alternative therapy for pruritus that is refractory to first-line therapies. Mirtazapine is believed to centrally reduce itch by antagonizing a2-adrenergic receptors [6,7]. Aside from having a wide therapeutic index, mirtazapine is rarely known to cause the initial anxiety and nausea associated with other antidepressants effective in treating chronic itch [2,8]. To assess the efficacy of mirtazapine for the treatment of chronic pruritus, we therefore performed a systematic review of the current literature using PubMed for English-language articles containing the words ("pruritus" or "itch") AND "antidepressant." The Preferred Reporting Items for Systematic Reviews and Meta-Analysis (PRISMA) flow chart is shown in Figure 1. All studies reported a reduction in itch intensity following the administration of mirtazapine. Collectively, these studies suggest the potential for mirtazapine to relieve chronic itch attributed to dermatological causes and malignancies (Table 1).

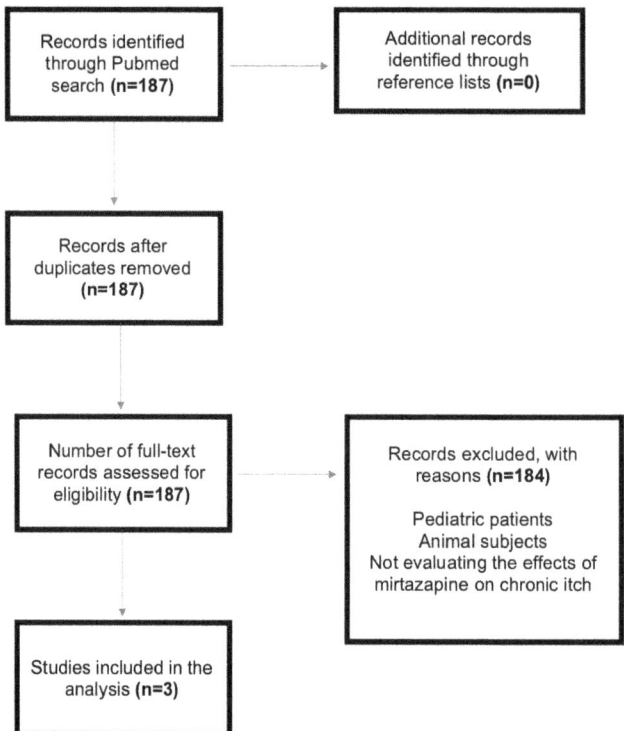

Figure 1. Preferred Reporting Items for Systematic Reviews and Meta-Analyses (PRISMA) flow-chart. *n*, number of articles; *Mirtazapine*.

Table 1. Summary of studies examining the effects of mirtazpine in treating chronic pruritus. * Determined based on the Oxford Centre for Evidence-based Medicine (CEBM) Levels of Evidence. *Mirtazapine*; CS, case series; CR, case report.

Grade of Recommendation *	Study Design	Diagnosis	N	Regimen	Degree of Pruritus Reduction	Reference
C	CS	Atopic dermatitis	2	15 mg mirtazapine every day for three months (first patient) and six months (second patient).	Both patients noted a "significant reduction" of nocturnal and daytime pruritus and improvement in sleep.	[7]
		Lichen simplex chronicus	1	15 mg mirtazapine every day for two months.	Patient noted a complete resolution of nocturnal pruritus and "significant reduction" in daytime pruritus.	
C	CS	Adenocarcinoma of unknown origin		15 mg mirtazapine every night until death.	The patient reported complete resolution of pruritus within 24 hours.	[2]
		Nodular sclerosis Hodgkin's disease		15 mg mirtazapine every night. After an unspecified length of time, the dosage was increased to 30 mg every night until death.	The patient reported 75% improvement in pruritic symptoms on 15 mg mirtazapine and complete resolution of itch on 30 mg mirtazapine.	
		Large B-cell lymphoma	4	15 mg mirtazapine every night. After an unspecified length of time, the dosage was increased to 30 mg every night and continued for an unspecified length of time.	The patient reported 80% improvement in pruritic symptoms on 15 mg mirtazapine and complete resolution of itch on 30 mg mirtazapine.	
		Advanced renal cell carcinoma		15 mg mirtazapine every night. One month later, dosage was increased to 30 mg and maintained at that level until death.	The patient reported complete resolution of pruritus on 30 mg mirtazapine.	
C	CR	Carcinoma en cuirasse	1	15 mg oral mirtazapine every night for an unspecified duration.	The patient reported a decrease in itch intensity from "200/100" pre-treatment to 2/100 twelve hours after starting mirtazapine.	[6]

There are several limitations to this review. Of the studies evaluated, most were case series or case reports. Larger, randomized controlled trials are still needed to draw definitive conclusions regarding mirtazapine's effectiveness in reducing itch. The studies included used a wide variety of outcome measures to evaluate itch intensity, which limits our ability to directly compare outcomes. Given the significant psychological burden of chronic pruritus, the placebo effect may have also affected perceived outcomes [9].

Mirtazapine is currently FDA-approved for the treatment of major depressive disorder. The main side effects of mirtazapine are heavy sedation, weight gain and hypercholesterolemia [10]. Mirtazapine is contraindicated in patients taking monoamine oxidase inhibitors (MAOIs) given the increased risk of serotonin syndrome [6]. Prior to prescribing mirtazapine, physicians should obtain a baseline lipid panel, liver function tests, and fasting blood glucose levels [11]. The FDA-approved starting dose for mirtazapine is 15 mg orally every night for the treatment of major depressive disorder (MDD) [7,11]. Physicians should counsel patients to report any signs of worsening depression or suicidal ideations upon the initiation of treatment or as a result of dosage changes. It is also advised that physicians schedule a follow-up appointment six-weeks after initiating treatment to evaluate for clinical improvement, drug reactions, or adverse effects.

In conclusion, mirtazapine may be an option for patients with chronic pruritus that is refractory to typical first-line treatments, but future randomized controlled trials are needed to determine the efficacy of therapy, optimal dosing regimens, and the types of chronic pruritus that benefit most from treatment with oral antidepressants.

Author Contributions: R.K., E.B. and S.G.K. conceived and designed the study; R.K. and E.B. conducted the literature review; R.K., E.B., J.G.Z. and S.G.K. analyzed the data; R.K. and E.B. prepared the original draft of the manuscript. R.K. and M.B. reviewed and edited the manuscript; J.G.Z. and S.G.K. supervised the analysis and writing of the manuscript.

Funding: This research received no external funding.

Conflicts of Interest: Shawn G. Kwatra is on the advisory board for Menlo and Trevi Therapeutics and has received grant funding from Kiniksa Pharmaceuticals. The other author(s) have no conflicts of interest to declare. The content in this manuscript has not been published or submitted for publication elsewhere. All authors have contributed significantly, and are in agreement with the content of the manuscript.

References

1. Dhand, A.; Aminoff, M.J. The neurology of itch. *Brain* **2014**, *137*, 313–322. [CrossRef] [PubMed]
2. Davis, M.P.; Frandsen, J.L.; Walsh, D.; Andresen, S.; Taylor, S. Mirtazapine for Pruritus. *J. Pain Symptom Manag.* **2003**, *25*, 288–291. [CrossRef]
3. Kaur, R.; Sinha, V.R. Antidepressants as antipruritic agents: A review. *Eur. Neuropsychopharmacol.* **2018**, *28*, 341–352. [CrossRef] [PubMed]
4. Boozalis, E.; Khanna, R.; Kwatra, S.G. Selective serotonin reuptake inhibitors for the treatment of chronic pruritus. *J. Dermatolog. Treat.* **2018**, *29*, 812–814. [CrossRef] [PubMed]
5. Boozalis, E.; Khanna, R.; Zampella, J.G.; Kwatra, S.G. Tricyclic antidepressants for the treatment of chronic pruritus. *J. Dermatolog. Treat.* **2019**, *6*, 1–3. [CrossRef] [PubMed]
6. Lee, J.J.; Girouard, S.D.; Carlberg, V.M.; Mostaghimi, A. Effective use of mirtazapine for refractory pruritus associated with carcinoma en cuirasse. *BMJ Support. Palliat. Care* **2016**, *6*, 119–121. [CrossRef] [PubMed]
7. Hundley, J.L.; Yosipovitch, G. Mirtazapine for reducing nocturnal itch in patients with chronic pruritus: A pilot study. *J. Am. Acad. Dermatol.* **2004**, *50*, 889–891. [CrossRef] [PubMed]
8. Davis, M.P.; Dickerson, E.D.; Pappagallo, M.; Benedetti, C.; Grauer, P.A.; Lycan, J. Mirtazepine: Heir apparent to amitriptyline? *Am. J. Hosp. Palliat. Med.* **2001**, *18*, 42–46. [CrossRef] [PubMed]
9. van Laarhoven, A.I.M.; van der Sman-Mauriks, I.M.; Donders, A.R.T.; Pronk, M.C.; van de Kerkhof, P.C.M.; Evers, A.W.M. Placebo Effects on Itch: A Meta-Analysis of Clinical Trials of Patients with Dermatological Conditions. *J. Investig. Dermatol.* **2015**, *135*, 1234–1243. [CrossRef] [PubMed]

10. Kuhn, H.; Mennella, C.; Magid, M.; Stamu-O'Brien, C.; Kroumpouzos, G. Psychocutaneous disease: Pharmacotherapy and psychotherapy. *J. Am. Acad. Dermatol.* **2017**, *76*, 795–808. [CrossRef] [PubMed]
11. Drugs, A. REMERON ®(Mirtazapine) Tablets. Available online: https://www.accessdata.fda.gov/drugsatfda_docs/label/2007/020415s019,021208s010lbl.pdf (accessed on 29 June 2019).

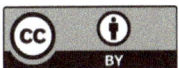

© 2019 by the authors. Licensee MDPI, Basel, Switzerland. This article is an open access article distributed under the terms and conditions of the Creative Commons Attribution (CC BY) license (http://creativecommons.org/licenses/by/4.0/).

MDPI
St. Alban-Anlage 66
4052 Basel
Switzerland
Tel. +41 61 683 77 34
Fax +41 61 302 89 18
www.mdpi.com

Medicines Editorial Office
E-mail: medicines@mdpi.com
www.mdpi.com/journal/medicines